D0707185

Water Therapy

Water Therapy

HOW TO USE HOME WATER TREATMENTS
FOR TOTAL HEALTH AND BEAUTY

Leon Chaitow

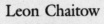

Thorsons
An Imprint of HarperCollins*Publishers*

Thorsons
An Imprint of HarperCollins*Publishers*
77–85 Fulham Palace Road,
Hammersmith, London W6 8JB
1160 Battery Street,
San Francisco, California 94111–1213

First published by Thorsons 1994
1 3 5 7 9 10 8 6 4 2

© Leon Chaitow 1994

Leon Chaitow asserts the moral right to
be identified as the author of this work

A catalogue record for this book
is available from the British Library

ISBN 0 7225 2862 0

Phototypeset by Harper Phototypesetters Limited,
Northampton, England
Printed in Great Britain by
HarperCollinsManufacturing Glasgow

All rights reserved. No part of this publication may be
reproduced, stored in a retrieval system, or transmitted,
in any form or by any means, electronic, mechanical,
photocopying, recording or otherwise, without the prior
permission of the publishers.

Contents

Amazing Facts about Water

If scientists were asked to invent a substance in which many other substances can dissolve (more things dissolve in water than are able to in any other liquid, making it very useful for transporting substances such as minerals to the body surface in hydrotherapy), which is almost universally available and inexpensive, which is non-toxic and non-irritating, which rapidly absorbs and holds a good deal of heat yet gives it up easily without cooling too rapidly, which can store energy and turn from liquid to vapour or to a solid, while being useful in all three states, they would undoubtedly smile, scratch their heads and say, 'Why invent it? We already have it – it's called water.'

Remember – at least 70 per cent of your body is water.

Water has the following major qualities, all of which we can use in hydrotherapy:

- Water is the most abundant compound (i.e. combination of elements – in this case hydrogen [about 90%] and oxygen [just over 10%]) on the planet.
- Water is extremely malleable – it can be made to touch almost every part of the surface of the body (and many parts inside as well). And when

absorbed in a towel or other material it can be moulded to all the contours and outer surfaces of the body to interact with the skin in remarkable ways. This makes it wonderfully useful for self-treatment.

- Water absorbs and gives out large amounts of heat, without changing its own temperature very much.

More of the amazing qualities of water will become apparent as the various applications are explained in the following pages. Some of the benefits come directly from the qualities of water itself, while others are due to the substances that you can add to it. Water is a powerful ally in the search for health and beauty.

1

What Water Therapy Offers You

Glowing good health feels good and looks good. And looking good – with bright eyes, soft and smooth skin, firm and flexible muscles – relates directly to being well, to being healthy.

Whether your aim is to retain a sense of healthy, energetic well-being, with all its outer and inner benefits (especially if you have noticed aspects of it slipping away slightly); or to restore or retain a highly efficient immune function, defending you against infection and toxicity; or to work towards regaining that ideal state of positive health – some degree of effort is called for. *But it does not have to be burdensome or unpleasant.* It can and should be pleasurable, fun – something that becomes an integral part of your everyday life.

Few would deny that we live in a period of constant and increasing environmental and social stress – and health (whether holding on to it or getting it back) depends on how well we handle the multiple physical and emotional stresses we face. Where we can't avoid negative factors, such as pollution in the atmosphere or having to live or work in situations that promote tension (avoidance is always the best form of defence), it makes sense to think about what we can do to defend our bodies and minds efficiently and, wherever possible, in ways that are pleasant. Water therapy – or hydro-therapy, to use its more technical name – is a highly effective and pleasurable way to achieve optimum health of mind and body.

While many of the health-enhancing methods and self-treatments you will find in this book relate to water and the multiple uses and potential benefits that this truly remarkable substance has to offer us, water treatments alone are obviously not capable of solving all our health problems. They do, however, offer means whereby we can help ourselves to well-being and to looking better as well. Water therapy can help us to retain or regain health, vitality, well-being and zest for life. It can also induce relaxation and ease pain.

For the very real reason that looking good helps enormously towards feeling good (and vice versa), much of this book is devoted entirely to just one aim – helping you to make the most of the assets with which nature provided you. The rest of the book deals with health, and in dealing with health there are two major areas of emphasis – keeping healthy and getting well again when there are health problems.

Although this book is mainly about water treatments for health and beauty, you are asked to remember that it is only when you are meeting *all* your needs (biochemical, structural, emotional, spiritual) that real health and glowing good looks will emerge.

Help Yourself to Health

Think about when it was that you last felt really well, on top of the world, full of energy, without a care or an ache or a health problem of any sort, when you would sleep easily and deeply, and wake refreshed and ready for anything. That desirable state of affairs can exist only when you are well nourished, emotionally balanced, getting enough (for you) exercise and providing yourself (or being provided) with all the many and varied requirements for health.

When, for whatever reason, you slip from that balanced state, there is only one way back to health, and that is by means of the self-healing mechanisms that we all possess. This sometimes needs help. Cuts heal, breaks mend, infections pass – usually without help – if your defence mechanisms are working well. Whatever treatment helps you along the way does just that – it helps you, it doesn't 'cure' you. *You* cure you.

In using water therapy you can help yourself to health. The more items you choose from the menu that this book lays before you – including good nutrition, adequate and ideal exercise, detoxification and relaxation, as well as water therapy – the better your body will be able to respond. So, if useful and pleasant water treatments can be combined with other health-promoting methods – such as relaxation, exercise, a balanced nutritious and delicious eating plan, and the luxury of massage – you have a potent recipe for increased good health.

The benefits that water therapy offers can be had by selectively drawing on the treasure-house of knowledge derived from traditional hydrotherapy, along with its modern versions, especially when the essential oils of plants and other safe, health-promoting natural substances are added to the water you are using.

Create Your Own Health Spa

A stay at a health spa is expensive. And while a fortnight, a week or even a weekend of being served delicious cleansing and nutritious food, of being regularly massaged with aromatic oils, bathed (in various ways), exercised, relaxed and pampered would undoubtedly be good for you, and would enable you to return to the battle refreshed and in a better state of both mental and bodily health, *it might be no more useful in the long run than having your car valet-cleaned and polished instead of having it serviced*. Because even if you can afford all that these remarkable places have to offer, probably the most they can do to combat the wear and tear of life is to provide a short-term respite from the onslaught of stress.

It makes a lot more sense to find a formula that can enable you to achieve these benefits *all the time*, whenever you need them, daily if necessary, and without the outlay of money that a stay at a health farm or spa or hydro demands. You could then give yourself the bonus of a periodic visit to a health spa to boost what you are doing for yourself – and to allow you to enjoy being pampered.

If you have a bathroom with hot and cold running water you already have the main ingredients of a home spa. All you need apart from that is a bit of basic organisation, some information (read on), some inexpensive materials (such as essential oils, herbs and towels), a bit of time for yourself and the determination to be well, healthy and full of zest. The rest should be fun.

A home spa is a common-sense approach which is within the reach of almost everyone. A home spa can be enjoyable, pampering, as well as health promoting, and you can use it in whatever way you want to. How much effort you put into making it a full and 'holistic' experience is up to you.

Ingredients for a Home Spa

The core of a spa is the water treatments, but to be truly effective these need to be linked to a balanced, wholesome diet, periodically interspersed with detoxification periods, and accompanied by gentle but regular exercise (including breathing exercises), relaxation and – if at all possible – massage. All these ingredients will be described in the following chapters, with water treatment taking centre stage. Your home spa will then be set up for health promotion, beauty and energy gains, first aid, and treatment of specific health problems.

A Warning Note

If you have a serious health condition – especially if this involves diabetes, cancer, or any other degenerative disease for which you are obliged to take regular prescribed medication – you should consult your qualified health-care provider before embarking on self-treatment involving dietary changes.

The water treatments are universally safe (if you follow the guidelines closely) except for a few that are contra-indicated for anyone with very high blood pressure, open skin lesions, specific allergies, or diabetes. All contra-indications will be listed in the text describing the methods.

Before looking at the history of water therapy and at current research into its uses for health, vitality and beauty – as well as how to use it safely and effectively at home – let's look at some of the reasons why we all need to take such self-help approaches seriously and at some of the methods which are available to you. Enjoy your journey into the wonderful world of water treatments.

2

How to Look and Feel Better

The normal functions of life produce toxins all the time, the waste products of metabolism formed as our bodies create energy, digest food, transport blood or work muscles. These toxins are usually efficiently eliminated or neutralised by processes involving organs such as the liver, kidneys, bowels, lungs and, most importantly, the skin.

The toxins are created more rapidly and cleared more slowly when we are stressed. For example, if muscles are held tensely they create and retain acid wastes. These acid wastes can be flushed away by exercise and fresh, oxygenated blood, and they can also be excreted through the skin as sweat. Or they can be retained in the tissues due to sluggish circulation and poor oxygenation due to inadequate exercise and breathing. If toxins are retained they become irritants and interfere with normal function. Reducing tension and performing regular exercise and deep breathing, as well as introducing methods for increasing elimination through the skin, will reduce part of your toxic burden.

All your organs of detoxification need to be well nourished in order to work efficiently: well supplied with fresh, oxygenated blood carrying adequate nutrient supplies and served by a nervous system that is working correctly. As we get older, and as we are exposed to a greater degree of toxicity and stress from many sources, so our ability to self-cleanse – to detoxify – becomes less efficient, as do our various supporting functions such as circulation and elimination. Because of atmospheric, water and food pollution we all now carry within ourselves a cocktail of chemicals derived from solvents, pesticides, food additives, petrochemical by-products and heavy metals. If we do not efficiently eliminate these toxins we retain the load of this undesirable debris stored in our tissues, mainly in the fat below our skin. This is added to daily by exposure to new toxic materials in our food, water and the air we breathe, not to forget any extra toxicity we create or acquire through infection or from certain forms of medication.

No one has a clear idea of just what damage all this is doing to us, especially if you consider the combination of these toxic burdens interacting as they do with the very real individual biochemical differences we are each born with. We also all have huge differences in our levels of nutritional, structural and emotional excellence or deficiency. Some of us handle the toxic load better than others, but in the end all of us are negatively affected – sometimes with profound consequences to the levels of health we enjoy or the sort and intensity of the illnesses we suffer.

Good News for Health

The need to tackle these toxic burdens before they actually show up as ill health has never been greater – the good news is that there is an enormous amount each of us can do to help ourselves. Not only can we ensure a balanced diet, but we can make sure we get enough of the right sort of exercise. We can also take care of that vital area which controls everything else – our emotional and stress coping functions. And we can work at regularly cleansing our system, with water therapy as a key part of this process.

Many scientists believe that in the future health care will have at its very core an absolute requirement for safe and effective detoxification procedures. These procedures can and hopefully will be started before our immune system and vital organs have started to decline in efficiency. A healthy immune system, efficient organs of elimination and detoxification and a sound circulatory and nervous system can handle a great deal of toxicity. Supporting these functions, organs and systems – either because we want to keep them well and efficient, or because they may have shown signs that they are not operating optimally – is one of the best arguments for regularly using water therapy along with other self-help methods such as improved diet and exercise patterns.

Water therapy is safe, effective and cheap, and we can do it ourselves. Not only does it work, and work well, but it is often very pleasant to use – quite simply it feels good and makes you feel even better. With water therapy we can look better, feel better and protect ourselves at the same time, all with a very small investment of time and at very little cost.

Before looking at the ways in which water treatments can boost your health, and considering the choices you have as to what you eat and how much time you give yourself for relaxation, it's worth assessing just what your current state of health is. So answer the questions on the following pages to discover your personal health profile.

Questionnaire
Do You Need a Home Spa?

There are several questions in this section to help you identify where to place the emphasis in your health and beauty campaign.

Obviously if we were all to eat a balanced diet and relax sufficiently and exercise enough, while carefully avoiding exposure to toxins, we would all be pretty healthy – but most of us don't and aren't. And to confuse the whole scene it is now well established that what makes a perfectly balanced diet for you may not suit me; that you might need a great deal more (or less) exercise to stay fit than I do; and that because of where and how we were born and raised, and our respective parents' health status, and the many different things to which we have been exposed since childhood, you and I might carry quite different toxic 'burdens' in our systems and be able to cope (or not cope) with stress in quite different ways.

If this is true (and research shows that it is), how could it be possible for us to have the same requirements for anything, whether this be food or rest or exercise? Clearly it would not, so it is important to identify what your particular need for detoxification is, whether you may be nutritionally deficient, or overstressed or underexercised.

The questionnaires on the following pages give guidelines only – they are not meant to take the place of responsible medical assessment or care. They provide evidence of

tendencies and possibilities, not certainties. If they raise
doubts in your mind please discuss these with a professional
health adviser. The real aim of the questions is to help guide
you in making choices between the many options that are
presented to you in later chapters.

Are You Nutritionally Deficient?

The following signs can indicate nutrient deficiency, which
can mean that the particular nutrient listed is not forming
a sufficient part of your diet, or that you are not absorbing
and/or utilising the nutrients you are eating. Whichever is
the case, advice from a nutritional counsellor, dietician, or
naturopath would probably be a useful first step in correcting
an imbalance of this sort.

DO YOU HAVE: POSSIBLE DEFICIENCY
  1 A poor sense of smell
    and/or taste   Zinc
  2 Hair which is falling out or
    breaks easily?   Protein
  3 A very red or sensitive
    tongue?   Vitamin B complex
  4 Whites of eyes which are
    slightly blue?   Iron and/or Vit. C
  5 Gums which bleed on
    cleaning?   Zinc and/or Vit. C.
  6 Cramps at night?   Calcium/Magnesium
  7 Cuts which heal only slowly?   Zinc and/or Vit. C
  8 Rough skin on elbows
    or knees?   Vitamin A
  9 Trouble seeing at twilight?   Vitamin A

DO YOU HAVE:	POSSIBLE DEFICIENCY
10 Red, greasy and scaly skin on the face or nose?	Vitamin B2
11 Seborrhoeic dermatitis of the face or nose?	Vitamin B6
12 Cracking at the corners of the mouth?	Vit. B2 or B6 or folic acid

A balanced diet (see chapter 3) will help to sort out this sort of imbalance naturally. Supplementation of vitamins should be undertaken after taking responsible advice from a health-care professional.

Do You Need to See Your Doctor?

If you notice

- an increased need to quench your thirst
- a much increased need to urinate
- unaccountable loss of weight
- increased appetite and excessive fatigue

there could be a tendency to diabetes and you should see your doctor as soon as possible.

If you

- become breathless on exertion
- have a tendency to swollen ankles
- get palpitations
- have pale lips and fingernails
- have a blue tinge to the whites of your eyes

you may be anaemic and should see your doctor as soon as possible.

Do You Need to Detoxify?

1 Do you drink more than one and a half glasses of wine, or one pint of beer, or any spirits daily? (YES scores 3 points)
2 Do you drink more than a single cup each of coffee or tea daily? (YES scores 3 points)
3 Do you eat or drink chocolate or drink cola more than once a week? (Yes scores 3 points)
4 Do you drink tap water or use it in cooking or when making drinks? (YES scores 3 points)
5 Do you eat smoked, preserved or barbecued foods more than once a week? (YES scores 3 points)
6 Do you eat mainly 'normal' (i.e. not organically grown) vegetables and fruit? (YES scores 3 points)
7 If you do eat 'normal' fruits do you eat the skin (apples, pears, etc.)? (YES scores 3 points)
8 If you eat 'normal' vegetables do you wash them well and scrub and peel root vegetables to eliminate chemical residues? (NO scores 3 points)
9 Do you eat mainly 'normal' (i.e. not free range) meat, poultry and eggs? (YES scores 3 points)
10 Do you eat foods more than once a week which contain colouring, preservatives or other additives? (YES scores 3 points)
11 Have you taken prescription medication for depression, anxiety or sleep disturbance for more than a month in the past year?
12 Have you had an amalgam filling in your teeth within the last year, or do you have more than two amalgams in your mouth?

13 Do you smoke, live with a smoker, or take 'recreational drugs'?
14 Do you live or work near heavy industrial factories, a main traffic thoroughfare, or in a double-glazed office environment, or are you regularly exposed to or in contact with toxic fumes or chemicals of any sort?

If you score over 12 in this, or answer YES to questions 11, 12, 13 or 14, you are in need of some of the gentle detoxification methods described in later chapters. We can *all* benefit from periodic detoxification whatever our present health status.

How Stressed Are You?

If you are currently stressed and not coping well with it you will answer YES to most of the following:

1 In stressful situations do you become edgy and nervous?
2 If you are in a stressful situation do you commonly get breathless, tight chested and find yourself sighing and periodically taking deep breaths?
3 When upset or angry do you go bright red in the face?
4 If you had to speak to a group or meet new people would you feel physically sick, vomit or have diarrhoea?
5 If you are waiting to meet someone, or are feeling apprehensive about something, do you sweat, get strange feelings in the stomach and/or get goose-pimples on the skin?
6 In the same situation as question 5 does your pulse

start to race or do you feel a pounding in the head?

7 If a sudden sound is heard do you get very startled and feel upset?

8 Do you grind your teeth and/or find yourself fiddling with your hands or fingers a lot?

The more YES answers to these questions, the more stress is affecting you right now and the more you need to learn to relax and let go.

People who cope best with stress of any sort have certain characteristics. If you already have most of these characteristics your need to do much about increasing your 'stress-proofing' will be far less important than if you lack the characteristics of good stress copers. The chances are that the more YES answers you gave to the questions above, the more 'a' answers you will give to the next four questions.

1 Do you
a) dread change and feel threatened by it, or
b) welcome change as a challenge, an opportunity for development?

2 Do you
a) find it difficult to get involved in discussion or socialising when you are in a room full of strangers, or
b) find yourself chatting comfortably and interacting with strangers?

3 Do you
a) feel that 'things' happen to you and your family which you cannot control or deal with, or
b) that life-events are at least partially within your control and/or that you can deal with events when they occur.

4 Do you
   a) feel that life in general moulds you and that what happens in your life is determined by fate, or
   b) that you can influence and have some control over your own destiny.

Obviously the more 'b' answers the better and the more 'a' answers the more work there is for you to do in learning to take charge of your life. Starting a home spa in which you are actually taking responsibility for your health and fitness is an excellent way to begin this process.

If you have a cluster of 'a' answers there is likely also to be a tendency towards frequent feelings of anxiety and nervousness, a sense of failure, poor self-esteem, lack of confidence, difficulty in concentrating or making decisions or easily expressing deeper feelings, and a tendency towards dwelling on either past or future events rather than on present time. As you practise deeper relaxation, improved breathing and improved dietary patterns, along with appropriate hydrotherapy measures, so you should become less anxious and self-critical and more self-confident, focused and decisive. Later chapters (especially 3, 4, 11, 12 and 13) will help you towards these goals.

Consider seeking professional counselling if there are major anxieties that remain unexpressed and unresolved.

Exercise and Lifestyle

How we structure our daily routine has a powerful influence on our health, and this includes exercise (or lack of it) and a host of less obvious factors which the questions below will help you focus on.

1 Do you work (in the home or out of it) for more than 40 hours a week?
2 Do you regularly work for more than 10 hours on any given day?
3 Do you spend less than half an hour over your main meals?
4 Do you eat quickly, not chewing adequately?
5 Do you get less than seven hours sleep in 24?
6 Do you spend some time, regularly, listening to relaxing music?
7 Do you regularly practise some form of relaxation?
8 Do you get at least half an hour's active exercise three times a week?
9 Do you enjoy a creative hobby (gardening, painting, music, etc.) and spend time on this regularly?
10 Do you perform some sort of non-competitive activity such as yoga, tai chi, cycling or swimming?
11 Do you have regular bodywork treatment for relaxation (osteopathy, massage, aromatherapy, reflexology)?
12 Do you get outside in the fresh air in daylight for at least half an hour each day?

The answers to questions 1 to 5 should be NO, and if they are currently YES you should try to modify the situation to turn them into NO answers over a period of time.

The answers to questions 6 to 12 should all be YES, and if they are currently NO you should try to modify them slowly towards YES.

3

An Unbalanced Diet – the Enemy of Health and Beauty

There are thousands of books on diet, so this chapter will be brief and to the point. If you intend to help yourself to health and glowing good looks then whatever you do with exercise, water therapy or relaxation will be only partially successful unless you also pay attention to your diet. It is no coincidence that spas focus on nutrition above all else.

Diet, Illness and Aging

One important and not very well understood aspect of how diet influences not just health but appearance as well involves some minute 'rogue' molecules called free radicals, which set up a chemical process known as oxidation, one of the major causes of aging and especially of one of its least attractive aspects – wrinkles.

When hair is bleached the change in colour is caused by oxidation. The same process takes place when metal rusts or tarnishes, when rubber perishes, when fats or oils become rancid or when a potato or apple turns brown when cut in half. It also happens inside you and me, all the time, because oxidation is one of the ways in which your immune system protects you from harmful bacteria. Your defence cells actually manufacture tiny amounts of hydrogen peroxide to kill them. But while oxidation can be a useful natural process, it can also be damaging. Oxidation is thought to be one of the main ways in which arthritis, hardening of the arteries and cancer begin, as well as being a major part of the aging process.

What Causes Oxidation?

Every atom (you and everything else on this planet are made up of atoms linked together into molecules) has in orbit around it minute negatively and positively charged electrons and protons. They are usually balanced in pairs, making them stable. For example, when one oxygen atom joins with two hydrogen atoms we get a water molecule, H_2O, a stable substance with no 'free' electrons.

If, however, we have two hydrogen atoms and two oxygen atoms joined together we get H_2O_2 (hydrogen peroxide, or bleach), which has free electrons and is therefore a free radical.

A free radical is dangerous because its free electron causes it to behave like a violent football hooligan, grabbing electrons from any passing substance with which it comes into contact. If a stable molecule has an electron ripped away by a free radical it becomes unstable itself, and it will then try to hijack an electron from somewhere else.

Free Radicals and Our Bodies

When our defence systems manufacture free radicals to kill invading germs, they do it in such small amounts that damage seldom results in our own tissues, so this is not the source of dangerous levels of free radicals. One source may actually be your own tissues! Much of the material that makes up your body cells consists of lipid or fatty substances and these, like all fats, are likely under the wrong conditions to become oxidised.

Another source of free radicals is heavy metals, such as lead and cadmium, which are found in polluted air and water and which we all have inside our tissues as part of our toxic burden. Other toxic substances that cause free radical activity include tobacco smoke (which has high levels of cadmium and other free-radical containing elements) and by-products of the petrochemical industry found in the air we breathe or in our water supply. When 'wrong' conditions occur (too much fatty tissue and/or heavy metal toxicity), free radicals are most active and the chain-reaction of oxidation begins.

Stopping the Damage

Oxidation starts and goes on until substances called antioxidants come along to quench the process, just like putting out a fire (which is itself an example of free radical activity on a grand scale). Violent free radical behaviour is therefore controllable by a 'fire brigade' made up of antioxidant substances. For example, when, in a smoke-filled room, your eyes start to sting, this is because of free radical activity irritating the surface of your eyes. The tears that follow contain glutathione peroxidase, a strong antioxidant enzyme, which quenches and stops this process.

It is always better to prevent something rather than trying to stop it once it has started. So a squeeze of lemon (antioxidant) on a cut apple stops it turning brown (oxidising), thanks to vitamin C. Antioxidants are what we use to rust-proof metal or stop it from tarnishing. They also preserve oils and fats in food from going rancid, and they can preserve us from the worst effects of the aging process.

Protection is therefore available from eating antioxidant-rich foods. Antioxidants are found most plentifully in fresh fruit and vegetables, which is one reason for the medical emphasis on high levels of them in our diets. Antioxidants include vitamins A, C and E, and a trio of anti-aging, protective enzymes – superoxide dismutase, catalase and glutathione peroxidase – found in young sprouting plants, many fresh fruits (especially papaya, mango, pineapple, kiwi fruit and berries) and salad vegetables.

We gain a lot of these enzymes by eating such foods, or by supplementing ourselves with freeze-dried juice from sprouting plants such as wheat, which is particularly rich in them. General 'insurance' supplementation of antioxidants is easy thanks to products that combine the best of them, including vitamins A, C, E and selenium. Powerful plant-based antioxidant enzymes, as mentioned above, are also available for those who wish to boost protection even more.

The best approach, of course, is to avoid contact with free radicals if possible – fresh air, clean pure water, no smoking – and to boost natural antioxidant intake through fresh food, preferably lightly cooked or raw. If you are really aiming for high-level well-being, energy galore and eyes and skin that express the inner health you have created, then a diet that provides all your nutrients in an easily digested form is your best approach. The detoxification diet outlined below gives you another opportunity to minimise the damage caused by oxidation. You should be able to build this into your normal routine without difficulty.

The Gentle Detox Programme

Before deciding to detoxify get advice from a health professional to help you select the degree of intensity with which you should apply the various methods available. If you are robust and vital a more vigorous programme will be appropriate than if you are unwell or your health is fragile. Are you well enough to undertake rapid and active detoxification or is it better to string the process out in order to do the job slowly? Whichever is better for you, the ingredients of the detox programme are the same – it's only the speed and strength of what is done that needs to be modified according to individual needs.

The following detox programme is safe for almost everyone, but do check with your health adviser first. *If you are a recovering drug user or alcoholic or have an eating disorder or are a diabetic, then do not apply these methods without asking professional advice first.*

Priority number one in detoxification is dietary. Over almost every weekend for a few months, and thereafter once a month at least, choose between the following detoxification diets.

Short Water-only Fast

This lasts for 24 to 36 hours, conducted over a weekend – starting Friday evening and ending Saturday evening, or just all day Saturday so that work schedules are not interfered with. Make sure that you consume not less than four and not more than eight pints of water during the day. On the Sunday have a raw-food day, with fruit and salad only, well chewed, plus as much water as you like.

Full Weekend Monodiet

Start on Friday night and go through to Sunday evening on a single food. You can have up to three pounds daily of any of a single fruit such as grapes, apples, pears (the best choice if an allergy history exists) or papaya (ideal if digestive problems exist); or brown rice, buckwheat or millet; or potatoes (skin and all), boiled and eaten whenever desired. You can eat up to a pound dry weight of any of the grains (made palatable by the addition of a little lemon juice and olive oil) or three pounds of potatoes daily.

Whichever type of weekend detox you choose make sure you rest and keep warm and have no engagements – this is a time to allow all available energy to focus on the repairing and cleansing processes of detoxification.

In between these weekend detoxification intensives, a milder midweek programme of detoxification will boost your health still more.

Midweek Detox Diet

Breakfast
Choose between the following:

- fresh fruit (raw or lightly cooked, with no sweetening) and live yogurt
- home-made muesli (seeds and nuts and grains) and live yogurt
- cooked grains (buckwheat, millet, linseed, barley, rice, etc.) and yogurt

DRINK
Herbal tea (linden blossom, chamomile, mint, sage, lemon verbena) or a lemon and hot water drink.

Lunch and Supper
One of these should be a raw salad with jacket potato or brown rice and either bean curd (tofu) or low-fat cheese or nuts and seeds. Or, if raw food is a problem, a stir-fried

vegetable and tofu meal, or steamed vegetables eaten with potato or rice together with low-fat cheese or nuts and seeds.

The other main meal should be a choice between fish, chicken, game or vegetarian savoury (a pulse and grain combination) and vegetables lightly steamed, baked or stir-fried.

DESSERTS
Lightly stewed fruit (add apple or lemon juice, not sugar) or live natural yogurt.

Season food with garlic and herbs, avoiding salt as much as possible. Eat slowly, chew well, don't drink with meals and consume at least two pints of liquid daily between meals. Also take one high-potency multimineral/multivitamin capsule daily and three garlic capsules, along with an acidophilus supplement for bowel detox support.

Additional Detox Support
The treatments described throughout this book will aid your detox programme. They include:

- Epsom salt baths or wet-sheet packs (see chapter 11 for details) – once weekly
- skin brushing to assist skin elimination function (see chapter 11) – daily
- stretching and relaxation exercises (see chapter 13) – daily
- if appropriate, brisk aerobic exercise (walking, jogging, skipping, rebounding, dancing, workout) – every day except during the fasting period
- massage and lymphatic drainage massage as often as available – twice weekly if possible

- use of appropriate essential aromatherapy oils (see chapter 9) – in baths or as part of massage
- breathing, relaxation and meditation methods (see chapter 4) – every day at least once for 10–15 minutes, twice would be better.

What to Expect

In the early days (the first few weekends) you could develop a headache and furred tongue – this is fine. It will slowly get less obvious as detoxification progresses. *Take nothing to stop the headache, just rest as much as you can.*

As the weeks pass your skin and eyes should become clearer (although your skin may get a bit spotty for a while), your brain sharper, your digestion more efficient, your energy levels should rise and you should regain a feeling of youthful clarity.

When your tongue no longer becomes furred with the weekend detox and headaches no longer appear, you can begin to spread these intensive detox weekends apart – three a month and then two a month and then maintenance of once a month. The in-between pattern can also be relaxed a bit, with the inclusion of a few 'naughty but nice' tasty toxins from time to time. By this time your internal detox system should be able to cope with such indiscretions – enjoy!

4

Calming the Mind

The ripple effect of anything positive or negative in our emotions reaches into how energetic or lethargic we feel, how enthusiastic or listless we are, how vital or empty we seem to others. And it shows – in body language and in appearance.

The difference between being bright-eyed, alert, purposeful and ready for action, and being dull, droopy, unresponsive and unenthusiastic about anything and everything can lie in as simple a factor as how well or badly you handle stress. The secret of coping with stress lies both in avoiding as much of it as you can and in learning to give your mind and body escape routes to relaxation in which balance can be restored.

There are a number of easily learned techniques, described below, which can help enormously in this direction, and any health and beauty strategy needs to include them. There is not a single health spa that does not have as a major part of its menu opportunities to unwind and relax, in both mind and body.

The various water-therapy measures listed in later chapters, combined with the use of essential oils and herbal infusions, the receiving of massage, regular pleasant forms of exercise and balanced nutrition all offer protection against the effects of stress. But they demand that one more ingredient be dealt with – your mind.

Relaxation Formula

There is a simple formula that you can use to check whether you are taking account of everything you need to do in order to achieve relaxation.

Diet
If you are to be really relaxed and able to cope with stress your diet should be nourishing, while your intake of 'tasty toxins' and stimulants should be as low as possible.

Muscular Release
It is important to find a way to release tension from your muscles. This might call for massage, stretching, exercise, water therapy or better nutrition. Muscular release is the first step towards calming the mind, because the mind cannot be calm if your muscles are tense. It also saves energy.

Full Breathing
Your breathing should be full and free. This can be achieved through massage, exercise, stretching, water therapy along with essential oils, and through the breathing exercises described below. Full breathing leads to better circulation and oxygenation and has specific effects on feelings of anxiety and being 'stressed out', since the body cannot relax or cope well with stress if it is poorly supplied with vital oxygen and nutrients.

A Calm Mind
Once you have achieved muscular release and full breathing you need to learn to still and focus your mind, so releasing

yourself from the constant internal chatter of daily events and anxieties. This calls for a form of meditation which suits you (see below). Meditation leads to a profound sense of being centred and at ease, which shows to those around you as your ability to concentrate and remember details is boosted and your whole being reflects calmness.

Creative Visualisation

And finally, once you have taken care of muscular tension and breathing, and your mind is still, you need to exercise it in creative visualisation and guided imagery – creating pictures in your mind – to round out your personal journey towards health and happiness. Depending on your belief system this can include spiritual dimensions and should certainly allow for growth in your personal sense of worth and usefulness.

To summarise: a good diet, muscular release, full breathing, mental calm and guided imagery – these simple steps *in this sequence* – can protect you from the worst effects of stress as well as allowing you to feel and look and function at your best, with energy to spare.

Recognising Stress

Are you feeling the effects of stress right now? You can easily recognise high stress levels when you show any of the following signs:

- being more restless or easily upset than usual
- difficulty in relaxing
- a disturbed sleep pattern
- sighing a lot or breathing more shallowly than usual

- difficulty in concentrating
- feeling on edge
- an almost constant sense of anxiety

So what is to be done if you are feeling the effects of too much stress? Part of the answer is to learn to reduce your anxiety level, which may be a lot easier than you expect. You can start in a number of different ways in order to achieve this.

1 Breathing
Begin by learning a simple traditional yoga breathing method. These techniques have been shown in medical studies to lower feelings of being stressed very quickly indeed.

2 Relaxation
You can use one of a great many methods of relaxation, some examples of which are given below.

3 Visualisation
You can use visualisation or guided imagery to produce even deeper levels of relaxation.

4 Sleep
Don't neglect getting enough sleep. Many of the techniques in this book will encourage you to deeper levels of sleep and you should not fight this. How much sleep do you need? We are all different – some people function very well indeed

on four to five hours daily, while you may need seven or eight. The only way to know is when you find yourself waking alert and full of energy – that's when you're getting enough of it.

Stress-Reducing Breathing Technique

There are many exercises to help improve breathing, but there is just *one* that has been shown in medical studies to be effective in reducing anxiety levels. This is an exercise based on traditional yogic breathing.

Before trying the exercise you need to take a look at your breathing 'equipment'.

The Mechanics of Breathing

Sit or stand in front of a mirror and observe your shoulders as you breathe deeply. Do they rise towards your ears as you inhale – even a little? If so, you are using certain muscles which attach to your neck, shoulders and upper ribs in a way that should only happen when you are, or have been, running. To use them when all you are doing is sitting or standing still shows they are overworking, and this will influence the mechanics of your breathing in a negative way.

To retrain yourself out of this habit (which is all it is) and help reduce the tendency it produces to hyperventilate (and therefore increase anxiety levels) you should do the following exercise, either separately from the relaxation breathing described below or as part of it.

1 Sit in a chair which has arms and rest your arms on the chair.
2 As you practise deep breathing, make sure your elbows

are firmly pressed downwards towards the floor, against the arms of the chair.

That's all there is to the exercise, since while pressing down with your elbows it is impossible to use the muscles that you were using previously, and you *have* to use the correct breathing muscles. Do this exercise at the same time as the rhythmic breathing described below, or at another time, until you can sit in front of a mirror and inhale *without your shoulders lifting towards your ears.*

Relaxation Breathing

1 Lie or sit comfortably and inhale *fully* while silently counting up to no more than three (ideally two). Translated into practical terms this means that you fill your lungs fairly quickly. *Counting is necessary because the timing of the inhalation and exhalation phases of breathing is critical in this exercise.*

2 Without pausing to hold the breath at all, exhale *fully* taking four, five or even six seconds to do so (count silently at the same speed as when you inhaled). All inhalation should be through the nose if possible, while exhalation can be through the nose or mouth. What is most important is that the breathing out must be slow and continuous. It is no use breathing the air out in two seconds and then simply waiting until the count reaches five or six before inhaling again.

3 Repeat the inhalation (two seconds) and the exhalation. The objective is that, in time and with practice, you should make the exhalation phase last for eight seconds.

4 Repeat the cycles of inhalation and exhalation for several minutes with at least six cycles per minutes.

Each cycle should eventually last 10 seconds – two in and eight out – although at first you may find that two in and three or four out is all you can manage.

By the time you have completed 10 or so cycles your sense of anxiety should be much reduced and you will feel relaxed and peaceful. Do this exercise every hour *if you are anxious*. Otherwise spend a few minutes doing it morning and evening – *and use it whenever you feel tension building up*.

Relaxation Technique
(Modified Autogenic Training)

There are a vast number of relaxation exercises, but one in particular seems to suit most people – so try it and see. It needs repeating daily for a week or more before you can judge whether it suits your personal needs. If other forms of relaxation suit you better, then use them, since anything that produces a reduction of muscular tension and anxiety is going to give you more energy and help you feel and look better.

Autogenic training is best learned from a fully trained instructor, but the following modified form is a excellent way of starting to learn to relax.

1 Lie on the floor or bed in a comfortable position, with a small cushion under your head perhaps, knees bent if that makes your back feel easier, and with your eyes closed.
2 Focus your attention on your right hand or arm and silently say to yourself, 'My right arm or hand feels heavy.' Try to *see* the arm relaxed and heavy, its weight

sinking into the surface it is resting on. *Feel* its weight. Over a period of about a minute repeat the statement several times, and try to stay focused on the *weight and heaviness* of your hand or arm. You will almost certainly lose focus as your attention wanders from time to time. Staying focused is part of the training in the exercise, so don't feel angry, just go back to the arm and its heaviness. You may or may not be able to sense the heaviness – it doesn't matter too much at first. If you do, stay with it and enjoy the sense of release, of letting go, that comes with it.

3 Next, focus on your left hand or arm and do exactly the same thing for about a minute.

4 Move to the left leg and then the right leg, giving each the same message that you gave to your arms.

5 Go back to your right hand or arm and silently say, 'My right arm is feeling warm (or hot).'

6 After a minute or so go to the left hand or arm, the left leg and then finally the right leg, each time with the *warming* message. If warmth is sensed stay with it for a while and feel it spread. Enjoy it. Again, try to keep your attention focused.

7 Finally, focus on your forehead and affirm that it feels cool and refreshed. Stay with this for a minute before completing the exercise.

By repeating the whole exercise at least once a day (10 to 15 minutes is all it will take) you will gradually find you can stay focused on each region and sensation (warmth, heaviness, coolness) for the full minute in each case. 'Heaviness' represents what you feel when muscles relax and 'warmth' is what you feel when your circulation to an area is increased, while 'coolness' is the opposite, a reduction in circulation for a short while.

You can use the new skills you have gained to focus on any area where you wish to create a positive change in your health. For example, 'I am calm and relaxed', 'My aching back is easing and relaxing', 'I feel full of energy', 'My skin is clear' and so on. When you are internally verbalising this sort of message you are in fact practising visualisation, especially if you can stay focused on the message and area and if you repeat the message frequently, several times a day.

Visualisation

To be most effective, visualisation should follow on from deep relaxation. Positive visualisation means using 'mental pictures', creating harmonious, uplifting and safe images – a flowery sunlit meadow by a sparkling river; a quiet beach scene; a favourite garden or room – to produce a profound state of contentment. You simply see such a scene in your mind's eye, and then imagine yourself there. The next stage is to employ your mind to encourage any particular health-enhancing state (peaceful tranquillity, energised well-being, relaxation, strength, and so on) you wish to develop and enhance.

Whatever visualisation image you construct it is absolutely essential that relaxation be achieved first. Visualisation adds just one more dimension to relaxation, allowing the mind to become involved more actively in achieving health gains.

Relaxation Massage

No discussion about relaxation would be complete without a mention of massage. Massage is wonderfully relaxing – it also achieves a number of very practical benefits including

- easing congestion away from muscles
- improving circulation – both locally and generally
- soothing and calming tensions

While it is possible to massage yourself up to a point in local areas such as the legs and arms (one-handed massage!), you need someone else to do the job properly. You need either to invest in a professional therapist – who might well come to your home – or train someone close to you to perform this most relaxing and bonding of treatments. You and your partner or a friend can exchange massage treatments – not aimed at 'curing' anything but simply and importantly at achieving a relaxing and calming effect with all the healing and energy saving that this can bring. There are classes for learning massage – designed for the general public rather than for training professionals – at adult education centres, and hundreds of massage schools also run classes for the public in 'wellness massage'.

Recent research has shown that people who learn to give massage achieve lower blood pressure and reduced stress levels themselves. So giving and receiving this marvellous touch therapy is highly recommended and should be a major part of your health and beauty maintenance programme. A weekly massage would be good, and every other day would be even better.

5

The History of Water Therapy

Ancient history records many cultures, including the ancient Egyptians, Greeks and Romans, the Chinese, Indians and Japanese, and the classical civilisations of South America and Mesopotamia, as using many different forms of hydrotherapy or water therapy. In more recent times, John Floyer, a doctor in Lichfield, England, who was born in 1649 and died in 1734, wrote a 'History of hot and cold bathing', which was published in the last days of the seventeenth Century and went into many editions and was translated into a number of foreign languages. The German version is said to have had a strong influence on Johann Hahn (1696–1773), who with his family developed the basis of modern water therapy in Silesia, where just a few years later one of the giants of early water treatment, Vincent Priessnitz (1799–1852), had amazing results when he treated people using his version of water therapy. He became famous and worked under government authority despite having no medical quali-fications, teaching hundreds of doctors his methods.

Many others followed, including Johann Schroth (1798–1856), who combined the 'water cure' with fasting. Most notable of all was Father Sebastian Kneipp (1821–1897), whose work lives on today in Germany where there are dozens of Kneipp Kurhause using modern techniques of hydrotherapy where patients can stay for residential care paid for under the national health system.

Kneipp used hydrotherapy alongside herbal therapy, diet, exercise and general 'hygienic' treatment (fresh air, sunlight, rest), setting the basis for the evolution towards the modern health spa where all these methods would become available for tired and stressed city folk.

In the UK great hydrotherapy centres such as those at Bath were developed and similar establishments mushroomed throughout Europe, most notably in Germany, Austria, Hungary, Czechoslovakia and later France. Other followers of Priessnitz, and later of Kneipp, travelled to the Americas, where they enthusiastically applied the methods that these pioneers had developed. The most famous of all American spas (and in its time one of the largest in the world, with over a thousand patients in residence at any time) was that which grew around Dr John Harvey Kellogg (1852–1943) at Battle Creek, Michigan. Dr Kellogg invented the cornflake breakfast in an attempt to wean his patients away from the high-fat breakfast eaten in the USA in the late nineteenth century. His book *Rational Hydrotherapy* was first published in 1901 and is still regarded as the best textbook on the subject ever written.

In the UK modern spa treatment uses hydrotherapy as one of its centre-pieces alongside fasting, dieting, manipulative methods such as massage, exercise, relaxation, fresh air and sunbathing. Stanley Lief DO (1892–1963) set the UK pattern for such establishments at Champneys, still the flagship of luxury spa treatment in the UK.

So the methods described in this book come to you via the work of Austrian, Silesian, German, French, American and British workers in the field of hydrotherapy. It is an honourable tradition which has been much researched in recent years with suitably impressive results. You can read about some of these in the next chapter.

6

Modern Research and Water Therapy

To many people the whole idea of using water to prevent or treat ill health is quaint and slightly ridiculous. This chapter should convince you that this is just not so. Whether preventing the common cold, improving fertility, 'curing' chronic fatigue, enhancing immune function, helping heart and circulation function or promoting the healing of extremely painful lesions, hydrotherapy has within the last few years been proven effective – without side effects and with hardly any cost.

The first two examples in this chapter of medical treatment using hydrotherapy are so dramatically effective, so simple to apply and so safe that there is nothing to stop you from copying the methods described unless you have a medical condition which makes this unwise, such as heart disease, high blood pressure, or any chronic illness requiring medication. The last two methods, however, are not meant to be copied by you. They are described for one purpose only – to impress you with how efficient and how simple hydrotherapy is.

This is 'low-tech' medicine – it relies on very specific responses from the body to the precise application of hydrotherapy, based on a predictable pattern established over the hundreds of years of observation of how water does what it does to the body, and of how the body responds to it. It is folk medicine brought up to date and much of it is available to you for home use for first aid, for general relief of many symptoms, and above all for improvement of well-being. These methods of water treatment are safe (so safe that self-treatment is almost always possible and desirable), predictable (no side-effects if you follow the very simple rules) and extremely cheap.

Apart from the impressive results of water therapy described in this chapter, there are often also other benefits such as greater energy, improved skin function and appearance, and of course our primary objective – better health.

Preventing the Common Cold

In 1990 the Hanover Medical School decided to re-examine some of Father Kneipp's methods which he maintained would help to prevent infection. If the old priest's claims were accurate this would mean that the body's defence system, its immune function, could in some way be made more efficient by the use of methods devised over a century earlier, using simple water treatments as described in his book *My Water Cure*, published in English in 1899.

Fifty medical students volunteered to be in the six month trial. Twenty-five of them followed the old Kneipp method of taking an early morning shower which, over a period of weeks, was made increasingly colder until after about three weeks the students were taking a two- or three-minute cold shower each day, except when they actually had a cold and for a week afterwards. The other 25 students took an early morning warm shower all through the study period.

Over the first three months there was very little difference between the two groups in the numbers of colds recorded or in the intensity and duration of the colds. But for the second three months of the trial the students taking cold showers had *half* the number of colds that the 'warm-shower' group had. And not only did the cold-shower students have fewer colds, but those that they did have were shorter (less than half as long) and far less acute.

Father Kneipp had suggested over a hundred years ago that regular cold showers would have a 'hardening' effect that would protect the person from infection. He was right. (For a fuller report on this study see *Physiotherapy*, volume 76, no. 4, pages 207–10, April 1990.)

'Curing' Chronic Fatigue, Boosting Immunity, Potency and Fertility, and Improving Heart Function

The results of important hydrotherapy research in London involving 100 volunteers were published in a four-page spread by *The European* on 22 April 1993. The Thrombosis Research Institute, which conducted the research, claims that the results prove without question the dramatic value of carefully graduated cold baths, and it is gathering 5000 volunteers for the next stage of the research.

The method used in this research programme is called Thermo Regulatory Hydrotherapy (TRH). The results showed that when applied correctly the effect of TRH was:

- A boost to sex hormone production, which helps regulate both potency in men and fertility in women.
- Renewed energy. Sufferers from chronic fatigue syndrome (ME) were found to improve dramatically: one person confined to bed 18 hours a day in a state of exhaustion experienced 'a new lease of life'. The

person is quoted as saying, 'From the first day I have regularly undertaken the hydrotherapy. With each day the feeling of wellbeing increases to such an extent that I can hardly wait for the next morning to arrive.'

- Improved circulation in people with cold extremities. Circulation is found to improve rapidly with TRH, along with levels of specific enzymes which help circulation.
- Reduced chances of heart attack and stroke because of improved blood-clotting function.
- Increased levels of white blood cells (defenders against infection).
- Reduced levels of unpleasant menopausal symptoms.
- Some of the volunteers found that their nails became harder and their hair growth improved.

And how was this achieved?

There are four stages to TRH and it is essential to 'train' the body towards the beneficial response by going through these stages in the order described. The only equipment needed is a bath, a bath thermometer, a watch and a bath mat. The bathroom should be a comfortable temperature – not too cold and not very hot. The temperature of the water should be between 12.7°C and 18.3°C – colder for hardy people with strong vitality and less cold for those who are more sensitive or frail.

Stage 1
Stand in cold water in the bath for between three and five minutes as your internal thermostat (a part of the brain called the hypothalamus) starts to respond. Do not stand still, but walk up and down in the bath or march on the spot. Be sure you have a non-slip mat in place if you try this.

Stage 2

Your internal thermostat is now primed, so you should now sit in cold water for another three to five minutes – up to your waist ideally – so that the pooled blood in the lower half of your body is cooled and further influences the hypothalamus.

Stage 3

This is the most important part of the programme, in which you need to immerse your entire body up to the neck and back of the head in cold water. *Gently and slowly* move your arms and legs to ensure that the slightly warmer water touching your skin (warmed by you) is not static, so that the cooling effect continues. This stage lasts between 10 and 20 minutes.

Stage 4

This stage is for 'rewarming', and as this takes place a warm, glowing sensation will be felt in various precise locations such as the chest, feet and between the shoulder blades. Give yourself a brisk rub down with a towel, and then do some active exercise for a minute or two, such as running on the spot, walking up and down, rebounding or skipping.

Caution

Thermo Regulatory Hydrotherapy is *not* recommended for anyone with well-established heart disease, high blood pressure or chronic diseases requiring regular prescription medication, unless their doctor has been consulted and has approved its use.

Helping Kidneys and Heart

Doctors at the Royal Infirmary in Bristol tested a traditional spa treatment of full body immersion for people with fluid retention, possibly due to kidney or heart disease. The volunteers for the trial had no such problems, as the doctors simply wanted to test the effects of the immersion on kidney and heart function.

The water used was that of the famous Bath spa, and the volunteers were placed in a seated position with water up to and covering their collar bones. The temperature of the water was neutral, not hot or cold to the touch, but close to body temperature. They stayed immersed for two hours, during which time blood and other samples were taken.

The results were as follows:

- Kidney function improved dramatically without any stress to the organ. The average weight loss due to fluid loss through urination after the immersion was over half a kilo – more than the weight of water consumed before and after the immersion.
- Sodium and potassium excretion increased markedly as a result of the immersion.
- The blood became increasingly less viscous (sticky) during the first half-hour of immersion, which is a useful effect for people prone to clotting.
- The 'cardiac index' – how efficient the heart is in its pumping – was increased by a 'highly significant degree'. In other words, the heart was able to pump a great deal more when in the water than when outside it. It pumped 4.6 litres a minute outside the water, increasing to 7.4 litres a minute when immersed, with *no* increase in pulse rate or blood pressure. This means that the heart pumped more efficiently *without strain,*

probably because the resistance it pumps against (the tension in the muscles and blood vessels, for example) is reduced by the pressure of the water.

When the doctors did the same tests using tap water, they got the same results.

The importance of this test to all of us is that the heart and kidneys can be safely helped by lying or sitting in water of body temperature (hot or cold water produces a different effect) for an hour or more. When this simple method is used to treat people with kidney and heart problems a dramatic release of retained fluid is experienced *without stress to the weak or sick organs,* as the next example shows.

In 1987 a 42-year-old male patient was treated using hydrotherapy at the Bristol Royal Infirmary for advanced cirrhosis of the liver, which had produced ascites (a huge swelling of the abdomen caused by fluid retention). The remarkable result was published in the *Journal of the Royal Society of Medicine,* volume 80, December 1987, pages 776–7.

The patient was given normal diuretic treatment for his condition and a low-salt diet, but this failed to produce any benefit over a two-week period. At that point the consultants decided to try a method that had been described in a classical text over 200 years before – immersion in water. The man, who had entered hospital weighing 84 kilos and had gained weight (fluid) despite the diuretic treatment, was placed seated in water up to his neck, at a temperature of 35°C, which is body heat, for two hours each day for the next six days. The results were dramatic and impressive.

Over the next few hours after the hydrotherapy immersion he lost 2 kilos in weight as his urine flow improved rapidly. With a combined use of hydrotherapy and the diuretic he was down to 76 kilos by day 19 – a loss of 8 kilos in six days, almost all of it fluid. By that time his ascites was gone, all swellings had vanished, and by following a low-salt diet and reducing his alcohol intake his condition stabilised.

The doctors stated: 'We suggest that the use of appropriate diuretics with water immersion is a safe and effective method of treating those people with cirrhosis with ascites who fail to respond to conventional treatment.' Two hundred years earlier a report had been published of a similar case: 'A scotchman in an ascites was cured. By his girdle which I saw fell six inches [he lost six inches around the stomach] in five days, pissing freely all the time.' (Sutherland, A., *An Attempt to Ascertain the Virtues of Bath and Bristol Waters,* Frederick and Leake, London 1764, pages 352–3.)

Note

Anyone with heart or kidney conditions should consult their doctor before trying to use this approach. Ask them to get (from a medical library) a copy of the report on this study, 'Observations on the effects of immersion in Bath spa water' by Dr J. O'Hare (and colleagues), published in the *British Medical Journal,* volume 291, 21–28 December 1985, pages 1747–51.

Healing Open Wounds

A painful and not much discussed problem affecting many people is that of anal fissures – cracked and ulcerated wounds near the anus, which are aggravated by constipation. Treatment is usually by means of expensive suppositories, creams and ointments, and sometimes by surgery. The traditional hydrotherapy treatment for this problem is usually a warm 'sitz' bath.

A Danish hospital decided to compare modern and traditional methods and monitored just over 100 patients over a three-year period to get a real idea of the benefits. Patients who had developed anal fissures for the first time were given one of three treatments: Lignocaine ointment (a pain-killer); Hydrocortisone ointment (an anti-inflammatory); or warm sitz bath and use of unprocessed bran (10 grams morning and evening) to help their constipation. The sitz baths comprised sitting in hot water (40°C) for 15 minutes morning and evening and wherever possible after every bowel movement. They could use the bathtub for the sitz bath or a plastic bowl.

The results? Let the doctors who did the study have the last word: 'Our findings show plainly that most patients with a first episode acute posterior anal fissure can be treated successfully with warm sitz baths combined with unprocessed bran, thus avoiding the use of anaesthetic and anti-inflammatory ointments. These other methods are less effective, more expensive and have unpleasant side effects.' This study was reported in the *British Medical Journal*, volume 292, 3 May 1986, in an article entitled 'Treatment of first episode acute anal fissure' by Dr Steen Jensen.

Hyperthermic Treatment

In chapter 13, which explains how hydrotherapy is used in spas and clinics, evidence of another amazing potential for hydrotherapy is given: how, by heating the body temperature using water, it is possible to deactivate cancer cells and many micro-organisms (viruses and bacteria) because they are heat sensitive. Hyperthermia involves using baths to raise the core temperature of the body to a level similar to that which occurs when you have a fever (in fact it is often called 'artificial fever therapy'). It is used for particular purposes such as cancer treatment and treatment of infections, including serious ones such as AIDS.

This method is *not* recommended for home use unless supervised by a competent and experienced health professional because it can be quite exhausting for the patient. Again the evidence is presented to impress you, to help you to gain a respect for the possibilities which hydrotherapy offers – many aspects of which you *can* safely use at home if you follow the simple and clear guidelines in this book.

7

How to Use Water Therapy Safely

Using water therapy at home gives you a range of simple and efficient ways of helping yourself to feel more energetic, to improve circulation, to tone skin and muscles, to be more relaxed, to improve sleep and generally to function more efficiently. The benefits of water therapy are far from superficial – there are very real health bonuses, such as boosting your immune system and improving the efficiency of the heart. Water treatments are also very effective at easing aches, pains, discomfort and stiffness, and they have wonderful cosmetic qualities.

There are different ways of using water therapeutically, and the different methods produce different beneficial effects.

The methods of water treatment that will be described in this book include

- heating compress (known in Europe as 'cold' compress)
- fomentation (usually hot damp applications)
- neutral bath (for anxiety reduction/pain relief)
- full sheet-pack (for relaxation and detoxification)
- ice-pack (for calming inflammation/easing pain)
- steam inhalations (for breathing problems/sinus congestion)
- alternating (or single) baths, sitz baths or local immersions (for circulatory stimulation/alteration)
- full baths of various types

Among the proven effects of specific types of water therapy
are:

- A reduction in general anxiety and feelings of being
  stressed, pressured and unable to relax. These can be
  helped enormously by use of a neutral bath or wet-
  sheet pack.
- Some methods reduce the sensitivity of nerve endings
  which report pain. Cold applications are good at this
  (using ice, for example), as are alternate hot and cold
  applications – wet towels can be laid on the area, or, if
  the painful part is small, such as a hand, this can be
  alternately 'dunked' in contrasting water for the same
  effect.
- A calming of inflammation, which often accompanies
  pain, can be achieved using alternating methods
  (cold/hot/cold) or cold alone for the appropriate length
  of time.
- When you use compresses and various contrast (hot
  and cold) methods you have several ways of reducing
  local swelling and congestion, such as occur with
  strains.
- Long cold applications, lasting more than a minute,
  reduce the speed of flow of blood to the area being
  treated, while hot applications encourage increased
  blood flow. By using alternations of hot and cold,
  circulation can be stimulated, improving skin and
  tissue tone and relieving the symptoms of poor
  circulation.
- Inactivity as well as overuse can reduce circulation to
  muscles and joints, leading to stiffness and sometimes
  pain, and this can be helped by simple methods such
  as contrast bathing, 'warming' compresses, cold
  douches, and hot and cold applications.

- Stiffness is eased when muscles relax. Hot applications can help this, as can 'warming' compresses (they go on cold but warm up because they are insulated) and alternating hot and cold applications or immersions.
- There are many ways of using different substances in water to assist in pain relief, including Epsom salt baths and a range of essential oils.
- Regular use of cold showers help reduce the incidence of colds and infection.
- Steam can be used with or without suitable aromatic herbs and oils to reduce the pain of chest and sinus congestion.

This chapter provides some guidelines to enable you to use these methods safely at home and reap their benefits. It also gives some important advice about conditions in which you should *not* use water therapy.

Guidelines and Applications

When you apply anything warm or hot to tissues the muscles relax and blood vessels open more widely. This causes more blood to reach those tissues. Unless there is activity (muscles contract and relax during exercise) or a cold application of some sort after this treatment, the tissues may then become congested. For this reason a cold application almost always follows a hot one.

When a short cold application is used it contracts the local blood vessels. This has the effect of decongesting tissues, and is rapidly followed by a reaction in which blood vessels open and tissues are flushed with fresh, oxygen-rich blood. Alternate hot and cold applications produce circulatory interchange and improved drainage and oxygen supply to the tissues, whether these be muscles, skin or organs.

Two important rules of hydrotherapy are that there should always be a short cold application or immersion after a hot one and preferably also before it (unless otherwise stated), and that when heat is applied it should never be hot enough to scald the skin and should always be bearable.

The general principles of hot and cold applications are that:

- short cold applications stimulate circulation
- long cold applications (more than a minute) depress circulation and metabolism
- long hot applications leave the area congested and static and demand a cold application to help restore normality
- short hot applications (less than five minutes) stimulate circulation but long hot applications (more than five minutes) depress both circulation and metabolism drastically
- short hot followed by short cold applications cause alternation of circulation followed by a return to normal

HOT is defined as 98–104° Fahrenheit or 36.7–40° centigrade. *Anything hotter than that is undesirable.* NEUTRAL applications or baths at body heat are very soothing and relaxing.

COLD is defined as 55–65°F or 12.7–18.3°C. Anything colder is very cold, and anything warmer is cool (66–80°F or 18.5–26.5°C) or tepid (81–92°F or 26.5–33.3°C) or neutral/warm (93–97°F or 33.8–36.1°C).

Reflexology and Water Therapy

Certain parts of the body, when heated or cooled, will have reflex effects on the circulation of distant areas. The main reflex connections are as follows:

- The skin of the feet and hands is reflexively connected with the circulation to the head, chest and pelvic regions (especially the bladder and reproductive organs, including the prostate in men).
- The skin of the lower breast bone is reflexively connected to the kidneys.
- The skin of the face is reflexively connected with the blood vessels of the head.
- The skin at the base of the neck area is reflexively connected with the mucous membranes of the nose (which is why something cold put on the back of the neck stops a nose-bleed).
- The skin overlying various spinal regions connects with the internal organs supplied by nerves from that spinal level (the lungs and heart with the upper spine; the stomach and liver with the middle spine; the bowels and abdominal organs with the lower back.
- The skin of the thighs, lower back and buttocks reflexively connects to the genito-urinary organs.
- The skin of the lower inner thighs connects with the prostate and uterus.

These reflex areas have various uses in hydrotherapy. For example, if you have a headache caused by cerebral congestion (too much blood in the head), a long cold application of more than one minute to the skin of the scalp would have the effect of constricting and therefore decongesting the vessels of the skull if the circulation could easily drain from the area – it might be impeded by muscular tension, which could be helped by gentle massage or relaxation. Other choices for congestive headaches would include:

- alternate hot and cold applications to the head
- cold application to the head and hot application to the feet
- ice-pack to the throat area to reduce circulation to the head
- cold application to the palms of the hands to reflexively decongest the head.

Caution

There are certain situations in which water therapy should be used with caution or not at all. For example, people with poor circulation or low vitality should not receive extreme contrasts of temperature. It is better for them to use a contrast of warm to cool rather than hot to cold applications.

For everyone, it is important not to use water therapy soon after a meal; leave it at least an hour and a half. *Diabetics should avoid any heat treatments to their legs.* Water therapy should not be used

- on extremely fragile skin
- where skin conditions are irritated by moisture
- over areas of numbness
- where there are serious circulatory conditions

although in these instances it is worth checking with a suitable health-care professional, because it could be helpful but might need special instructions.

8

Creating Your Own Health Spa

We are all individuals with unique characteristics and needs, and if you are to get the best out of your home health spa it is important that you devise a pattern of home care, whether for beauty or health or both, that suits your own needs, your own requirements. The whole process should be fun and not a burden or it could become self-defeating and add to your stress levels. Time is needed, and a personal space with special qualities.

Creating a Healing Space

Sound

Your personal health spa needs to include a variety of relaxation aids and an important one is sound. You should invest in some tapes of appropriate music and sounds, such as birdsong, forest sounds, whales singing – anything you find calming. You can also buy – or obtain from your local public library – tapes that talk you though various forms of relaxation, and some books contain 'scripts' that you can record for yourself to help you through relaxation and meditation processes. Sometimes hearing your own voice is more comforting than hearing someone else – it is a very personal matter. Although this voyage of discovery into your own inner space is one you need to take alone, it may help to have guidance from books and tapes at first.

Colour

The influence of colour on our mood is very strong indeed and if you can you should use colours to make your home spa as restful as possible. To some extent the choice of which colours relax or energise you will be a very personal matter. There are, however, general rules that seem to apply to all of us.

- blue and turquoise are calm colours and are 'cooling'
- green tends to be neutral, and while it is said to represent balance, it can make you feel lethargic
- mauve and violet have spiritual and balancing influences – they are calming and peaceful
- red is stimulating and warming but can be irritating and oppressive
- pink is often said to be extremely tranquillising and like mauve is associated with spirituality and calmness
- white is the colour of purity and some people find it calming while others are influenced negatively by white walls
- yellow and orange can be oppressive and irritating
- browns and beige colours are warm and protecting

So make your choice for the colours that will make your personal space as restful as possible.

Light

Full-spectrum light or sunlight is vitally nourishing to us and you should try to spend some time each day outside – if not in direct sunlight at least exposed to light without any glass (windscreens, windows, spectacles, etc.) between you and daylight. For your home spa try to get hold of full-spectrum light sources (bulbs or strip lighting) which will more or less replicate the spectrum of colours provided by the sun.

Take care over the placement of light so that your home spa is not too bright or too gloomy, and so that it is a welcoming and pleasant place to be.

Air

The selective choice of plants enhances air quality and beautifies any room. This is particularly necessary in modern homes, where many chemicals are found in carpets, curtains, furnishing, insulating materials, paints, and so on. Plants such as allaomena, syndonium, philodendron and spider plants all do a marvellous job of absorbing toxic fumes.

An ioniser, which costs very little, will add the benefits of negative ionisation to the air quality of the home health spa you are creating. It pumps out negative ions, which energise and stimulate us positively, and it balances the tendency in most modern homes for there to be too many positive ions, which make us feel lethargic and washed out.

And of course there is no substitute for getting out into the real fresh air as often as possible – daily, if you can, for a walk or just to sit and think.

By carefully combining plants and natural materials such as cotton, wool, silk, wood and clay with appropriate colours, sounds and light, you will create a magical place for yourself.

Making Time for Health

Relaxation

There are few things in life more important than feeling at peace with yourself and with your environment, including your relationships and your work. The fact is that we need to feel good about ourselves and those around us to function well, to feel well and to be at our best. So make sure that you give yourself some time each day to reflect, relax and unwind. This is the time for some form of relaxation or meditation. A daily 10-to-15-minute period is needed for this to be effective in positively influencing your life (see chapter 4). A weekly massage can also be wonderfully effective in helping you to relax.

Exercise

Also give yourself regular time for exercise. This should include active exercise such as walking, dancing, skipping, swimming or sport, always within the levels of your current fitness status (see chapter 13 for a method of measuring how 'fit' you are). It should also involve stretching type exercise (see chapter 13) for a balanced approach. Twenty minutes of active exercise three times a week and 10 minutes of stretching exercise daily are ideal.

Using your Home Spa

If you add to these demands on your time the exciting possibilities that the home spa offers you, you need to consider at least a further hour or two each week. This adds up to

Relaxation	2 hours per week
Massage	1 hour
Active exercise	1 hour
Stretching exercise	1 hour
Home spa	2 hours

It isn't really a question of whether you can afford the time to give yourself six or seven hours a week in which to take care of your most basic inner needs – it is more a question of whether you can afford *not* to do so! And the busier you are with work or family, the more important it is to make the time to look after yourself.

Of course, if you want to devote some of that time, or additional time, to use the home spa to enhance yourself cosmetically, that will also be beneficial. There is ample evidence from medical research to show that self-esteem, or how we feel about ourselves, has a strong influence on our well-being. So if your health can be helped by looking after your beauty requirements, then don't feel this is selfish or over-indulgent. In any case, you have the right to indulge yourself if you wish – to enjoy a massage, to float away cares in an aromatic bath, to lose yourself in deep relaxation and to use whatever safe and effective home treatment methods you want to in order to enhance and heal yourself.

What Else You'll Need

Among the other requirements for your home spa which you should start to accumulate are the following. All items listed are important, but those marked with a double asterisk are items which are essential if you want to follow the self-treatment ideas in later chapters.

For Your Bathroom or Bedroom

** a bath thermometer
** essential oils (see chapter 9)
** liquid moor (a peat-like substance) and mud (see chapter 10)
** dried herbs for bathing and for drinking as tea
** a skin brush (natural bristle) and a loofah or bath-mitten
** two large plastic bowls
** a non-slip bath mat
** towels, plastic sheeting, blankets, old cotton sheeting (some of this needs to be suitable for cutting into small squares or strips for compresses and packs)
** a shower head which can adjust to give different pressures/jets
** Epsom salts (commercial), sea salt
** a floor mat or futon or thin foam mat for floor exercises and relaxation
** a skipping rope or a rebounder (mini-trampoline)
 * bathroom scales
 * suitable spoken and sound or music tapes for relaxation and imagery and a portable player for use in the bathroom or bedroom
** an ioniser for use in the bathroom or bedroom
 * a nebuliser (to vaporise essential oils)
 * a vibrator/hand massager

For Your Kitchen

A juice extractor and lots of fruit and vegetables and spring water.

9

Essential Oils and Their Uses

The selection of oils described below all have beneficial properties. *None are meant to be consumed,* although many of the herbs from which the oils are derived can be consumed as teas to treat the conditions indicated as a first aid measure, provided the causes of the condition are also being dealt with appropriately. The oils are applied by rubbing them onto the skin or using them in the bath and, because of their aromatic qualities, by inhalation.

The use of essential oils as listed below is derived from the experience of many aromatherapists and herbal practitioners, and they are safe to use as indicated. The oils described here include the most useful and popular ones for self-massage or for adding to baths, but there are dozens more to try if you want. They can be used to alleviate very real health problems or just to help you feel better or, in a few cases, to look better – choose according to your personal needs.

When oils are to be used for massage they are seldom employed 'neat'. They are almost always added to a 'carrier' oil which is neutral and acts as a transport medium to get the essential oil to your skin without irritating it. Carrier oils can be derived from soy, sesame, almond, avocado, wheatgerm ('vitamin E oil', which helps preserve the oils from oxidation), sunflower or safflower (these last two are lighter oils and may not suit a dry skin). Most professional aromatherapists use a mixture of carrier oils before adding the essential oils. For example, four ounces of carrier oil (the standard amount) could be made up of two-thirds soyabean oil plus one-third sesame oil. If your skin is very dry, then a third each of soya, almond and avocado would be a better carrier mixture. When being added to a bath the oils are used neat in the running water which disperses and mixes them.

Store essential oils, individually or in combinations, in clean glass containers (dark if possible) away from light, tightly capped.

Basil

Antiseptic, antidepressant and a tonic for the digestion. On its own it can be used to treat weakness, physical and mental fatigue, headaches, nausea, tension, faintness and depression. Combined with neroli (six drops of each in four ounces of carrier oil for massage or 10 drops of each in a bath) it can relax you when you are tense, anxious or depressed.

Bay

Antiseptic, tonic and decongestant. On its own it can be used to treat colds. Use it with lavender for massage if there is hair loss (six drops of each in four ounces of carrier oil).

Chamomile

Soothing, sleep enhancer, digestive and general tonic, pain reliever and antibacterial. It can be used on its own to treat sleep and digestive disturbances, skin conditions, neuralgia, and inflammation. It soothes tired and irritated eyes when used as a compress or eyewash.

Combine it with rosemary for massage in cases of rheumatic pain (six drops of each in four ounces of carrier oil) or 10 drops of each in a bath for aches and pains of arthritic origin. The same combination, in carrier oil, can be used for migraine relief – massage the head, neck and abdomen. Together with basil (six drops of each in four ounces of carrier oil) it can treat indigestion if it is massaged into the solar plexus area. Used with marjoram (six drops of each in four ounces carrier oil) and massaged into the abdominal area and low back it can help menstrual cramps. It can also be used with cypress for haemorrhoids, and with lavender for sunburn.

Clove

Antiseptic, a stimulant for mind and body, and a reliever of spasm and pain. Used alone it can be helpful for infections, general tension and weakness. It makes a good mouthwash (2 drops in a tumbler of water) and is magical as a reliever of toothache when applied neat (in very small amounts on the tip of a cotton-wool stick) to the offending tooth or gum. Used with lemon it is an effective insect repellant.

Cypress

Astringent, antispasmodic, tonic and useful as a deodorant. It can be used alone to treat rheumatic and muscular conditions, coughs, flu and nervous tension.

Combined with lemon oil, a drop of the mixture is applied neat to acne spots and skin discolouration. It can be used with juniper for cellulite: either 10 drops of each in four ounces of carrier oil for massage into the affected area, or 20 drops of each in a warm bath.

Combined with chamomile – 20 drops of each in hot water for a sitz bath for 10 minutes – it is effective in treating haemorrhoids.

Combined with lavender – 20 drops of each in warm water or massage with six drops of each in four ounces of carrier oil – it is helpful for menopausal problems or for general nervous system treatment.

Together with geranium – 10 drops of each in four ounces of carrier oil – it can be used to gently massage over varicose veins, always massaging towards the heart.

Eucalyptus

Antiseptic, stimulant, insect repellant. It can be used alone to treat flu, sinus infections, laryngitis, breathing problems and coughs, rheumatism and open wounds.

Use it with sandalwood – add 10 drops of each to a bath – for arthritis and rheumatism, or the same combination in a strength of six drops of each in four ounces of carrier oil for massage onto the back and abdomen during urinary infections. It is effective with pine to treat coughs and bronchitis: use 10 drops of each in four ounces carrier oil for chest massage; or 20 drops of each in a hot bath; or 20 drops of each in a bowl of hot (steaming) water – place your face over this, cover your head with a towel, and inhale the vapour for sinus problems.

Combine it with lavender – six drops of each in four ounces of carrier oil – for massaging your abdomen and back when you have a fever, or for massaging into the temple area during severe headaches. The same combination can be applied to the head during a fever – use 10 drops of each in a bowl of tepid water, soak a hand towel and hold it to the head. With geranium it is a useful insect repellant.

Geranium

Tonic and stimulant of adrenaline, astringent, insect repellant and pain reliever. It can be used alone for neuralgia, slow healing of wounds and burns, and for poor circulation. It acts as a skin tonic.

Combined with rosemary – six drops of each in two ounces of carrier oil – it can be massaged into the abdomen, back and neck for fatigue. Or use 20 drops of each in a bath for a 15-minute soak, or eight drops of each in hot water for a foot bath (10 minutes) when very tired. Use it with eucalyptus – 10 drops of each in four ounces of carrier oil – as an insect repellant. Combine it with cypress for varicose veins.

Juniper

Nerve tonic, diuretic, and digestive aid. It is used alone to treat indigestion, nervous conditions, fluid retention, rheumatism and some skin conditions (it is antifungal).,

Combine it with cypress for cellulite – 10 drops of each in four ounces of carrier oil for massage, or 20 drops of each in bathwater for a 15-minute soak.

Together with marjoram – six drops of each in four ounces carrier oil – use it for abdominal massage if constipated. Mix six drops with the same amount of lavender in four ounces of carrier oil for massage if fatigued, or 20 drops each of juniper and lavender oil in a warm bath for haemorrhoids.

Together with thyme – either six drops of each in four ounces of carrier oil for abdominal massage, or 20 drops of each in a hot bath for ten minutes – it can help treat urinary tract infection. Combine it with rosemary to treat gout – either six drops of each in four ounces of carrier oil for gentle massage of the affected area, or 10 drops of each in cool or tepid water for a foot bath.

Lavender

Antispasmodic, antiseptic, general restorative, insect repellant. It can be used alone to treat nervous problems and skin lesions such as burns, wounds and acne. It makes a useful douche. Use a few drops neat on minor burns (although always call a doctor if burns are serious). Use it alone – 12 drops in four ounces of carrier oil for temple, head and neck massage – to treat headaches, or alternatively use 20 drops of oil in a bath for the same problem. It can be used together with thyme – three drops of each into two tablespoons of carrier oil – to treat insect bites; or lavender can be used alone, neat, on these; or use 10 drops each of lavender and thyme in a warm bath for same problem.

Combine it with vetiver – six drops of each in four ounces carrier oil – for back, abdomen and neck massage if anxious or tense.

Use it together with sandalwood and rose – six drops of each in four ounces carrier oil (combine soya, almond and avocado in ratio of 2:1:1 plus a spoonful of wheatgerm oil) – for very dry or chapped skin; with chamomile – 20 drops of each in a tepid (bodyheat) bath – for sunburn; with juniper for fatigue or haemorrhoids (bath or massage); with eucalyptus for fever (bath or massage); with bay for hair loss; and with cypress for menopausal or nervous problems.

Lemon

Tonic, antiseptic, diuretic, insect repellant. It can be used alone to treat rheumatic problems, digestive upsets, gout, fluid retention, poor skin tone. Use it with cypress, neat, on spots.

Combine it with clove oil – 10 drops of each in four ounces of carrier oil – as an insect repellant.

Marjoram

Stimulant and tonic. Combine marjoram with ylang-ylang
– six drops of each in four ounces of carrier oil – for massage
in cases of depression. Use it with juniper for constipation,
and with chamomile for menstrual cramps.

Neroli

Antidepressant, antiseptic, digestive aid, sedative, aphrodisiac. Used alone it can treat depression, insomnia and
nervous tension, digestive upsets and lack of sexual interest.
It is a skin enhancing agent. Use it together with basil for
bath or massage in cases of anxiety, tension or depression.

Peppermint

Stimulant for the nervous system, digestive aid, antispasmodic, pain reliever, insect repellant. Use it alone to treat
fatigue, indigestion, migraine and breathing problems,
including asthma.

Use 10 drops in four ounces of carrier oil for massage of
the base of the skull, the temples, neck and abdomen, or 20
drops of oil in a bath, to treat headaches. For indigestion,
massage the abdomen with 12 drops in four ounces of carrier
oil.

Pine

Antiseptic, diuretic and tonic (stimulates adrenaline
production). It is used alone to treat infections, fluid
retention, rheumatic conditions, coughs, colds and fatigue,
and together with eucalyptus for bronchitis, coughs and
sinus problems.

Rose

Antibacterial, antidepressant, aphrodisiac, astringent, sedative, tonic for the heart and liver. It has specific influences on the female reproductive organs, especially the uterus. Alone it is used to treat depression, poor sex drive, headache, nausea and insomnia, as well as being useful for douching and as a skin tonic. Use it with lavender and sandalwood for massage of dry and chapped skin.

Rosemary

Stimulant of hormones from the adrenal glands, antiseptic and decongestant. Applications on its own include treatment of colds and infections, rheumatic and gout-related conditions, burns and sores on the skin, fatigue and excess fat in the tissues.

For headaches, use 12 drops in carrier oil (four ounces) for head and neck massage, or 20 drops of oil in bowl of hot steaming water for inhalation.

Combine it with sage – six drops of each in carrier oil – for abdominal massage to treat nervous system problems, or use 20 drops of each in a bath for the same problem. Rosemary can be used together with chamomile for migraine headache, arthritis and rheumatism – either massage or a bath. Use it with thyme – six drops of each in four ounces of carrier oil – for abdominal massage if constipated, and with juniper for gout.

Sage

Tonic, antiseptic, diuretic, with influences on the female reproductive system and blood pressure. Alone it is used to treat nervousness, fatigue, chest complaints, menopausal problems, low blood pressure, and it is useful as a douche.

Use it together with rosemary for nervous system problems and with chamomile in menopausal problems.

Sandalwood
Antiseptic, aphrodisiac and tonic. It is used alone to treat bronchitis, urinary infections, impotence and fatigue; with eucalyptus for rheumatic and arthritic pains, and also for bladder and kidney problems; and with lavender and rose for dry skin.

Thyme
General stimulant, antiseptic, antispasmodic and neutraliser of snake venom. It is used alone to treat tiredness, digestive problems, infections, rheumatic conditions, inflammation of the skin, intestinal parasites and snakebite. It is effective with lavender for bites and stings.

Vetiver
This is a calming agent and is used to treat anxiety and nervous conditions. Combine it with lavender for anxiety and tension.

Ylang-Ylang
Sedative, antiseptic, aphrodisiac. Its use alone is for treatment of high blood pressure, intestinal infections and impotence. Use it with marjoram for depression.

Summary of Conditions and Appropriate Oils

Acne – cypress, lemon, lavender

Anxiety – basil, lavender, neroli, vetiver

Arthritis – chamomile, eucalyptus, rosemary, sandalwood

Bites and stings – basil, lavender, marjoram, thyme

Bladder problems – eucalyptus, juniper, sandalwood, thyme

Bronchial problems – eucalyptus, pine, sandalwood

Burns (not serious ones) – lavender

Cellulite – juniper, marjoram, rosemary, thyme

Chronic fatigue – geranium, juniper, lavender, rosemary

Colds – eucalyptus, pine, sandalwood

Depression – basil, marjoram, neroli, ylang-ylang

Dry skin – lavender, rose, sandalwood

Fever – eucalyptus, lavender, peppermint

Gout – juniper, rosemary

Haemorrhoids – chamomile, cypress, lavender, juniper

Hair loss – bay, lavender

Headache – chamomile, lavender, peppermint, rosemary

Indigestion – basil, chamomile, peppermint

Insect repellant – clove, eucalyptus, geranium, lemon

Menopausal problems – chamomile, cypress, lavender, sage

Menstrual cramping – chamomile, cypress, marjoram, sage

Migraine headaches – cypress, lavender, rosemary, sage

Rheumatism – chamomile, eucalyptus, rosemary, sandalwood

Sinus problems – cypress, eucalyptus, pine

Sunburn – chamomile, lavender
Varicose veins – cypress, geranium

Essential oils are widely available from pharmacies and health-food stores.

10

The Therapeutic and Beauty Uses of Moor, Mud and Clay

'Mud, mud, glorious mud, nothing quite like it for cooling the blood' . . . well maybe for a hippo, but what about you? The truth is that mud is a most amazing conglomeration of ingredients and it can be remarkably health enhancing – when used correctly. In this chapter we will look briefly at just three of the most researched and useful examples of mud, clay and peat, from Austria, Israel and France – there are many others.

Austrian Moor Products

Analysis of the extraordinary 'Moor' mud-like substance from Austria ('Neydharting Moor') shows that it includes an enormous variety of organic and inorganic minerals, oils, proteins, wax, resins, saturated and unsaturated fats, useful acids, natural antibiotics and vitamins.

Is this material peat? The Austrians say categorically no – peat, they explain, is the product of decaying trees which have been submerged in water for thousands of years. In the absence of air, the trees rot down and the end result is largely cellulose from wood fibre.

Moor, on the other hand, is the result of chemical, biological and biochemical changes in medicinal herbs and other plants including their roots, leaves, stalks, blooms, fruits, seeds and tubers. In the Austrian Moor products over 1000 different plants have been identified, 300 of which have medicinal value, and 200 of which have been extinct for over 500 years. These medicinal plants, with their unique elements, are preserved forever in the Moor, especially their trace elements, vitamins, plant hormones, plant antibiotics (to protect the plant against infection) and unique plant oils and wax.

It is estimated that Neydharting Moor material is around 20,000 years old and its use therapeutically dates back to before Roman times when the Celts first used it in 800 BC. The sixteenth-century physician Paracelsus wrote of its value, and the 'Moor Cure' was taken by King Louis XV and his Court, as well as by Napoleon and Josephine.

Modern research has now shown it to have enormous therapeutic value. It is an astringent, it is absorbent of toxic body wastes, acid balancing (ion-exchanging) and anti-inflammatory. The various ingredients of Moor penetrate the skin, helping its tone and circulation, as well as entering the body itself with wide-ranging influences.

Moor Beauty Products

NEYDHARTING MOOR LIFE SOAP
maintains skin acidity at its optimum level and is ideal for normal cosmetic use and for sensitive or damaged skin.

NEYDHARTING MOOR LIFE CLEANSING AND TONING LOTION
is ideal for either oily skin or dry and sensitive skin. It actively discourages acne and enhances skin tone, helping to restore and maintain skin acidity (pH) levels. There is also a Moor Face Cream and Body Cream for those who want to have the widest range of these remarkable products.

NEYDHARTING MOOR LIFE MASK
is made up of the essence of 20,000-year-old flowers, plants, grasses and herbs. Its essential oils and lipids penetrate easily into the skin and have a cleansing and rejuvenating effect. It is unperfumed and perhaps not too glamorous when on as a mask – but the results are what counts. The way to use it is as follows. Wash your face using Moor soap. Place a little of the Mask material into an egg cup and add a teaspoon of water. Mix until the material 'hangs' on to the skin of your fingers, not slipping off too easily. Apply the paste to the face with fingers or a brush and leave it on for three minutes if you have dry skin or up to eight minutes if you have 'problem' skin. Wash the face mask off with warm water and apply the Moor cleansing and toning cream, followed if you wish by the Moor face cream. This process is recommended once a week for normal skin, and daily for up to three weeks and twice a week thereafter for problem skins.

Additional beauty products from Neydharting Moor include shampoo, hair tonic, toothpaste, mouthwash and massage oil.

Moor Health Products

MOOR LIFE BATH
is taken at body temperature (a neutral bath, in other words) for about 20 minutes. The liquid ingredients are a mix of water and the Moor extract. No washing takes place in these baths – just lie and relax, and when leaving the bath pat yourself dry. The material will continue to be active for hours after the bath. The indications for using a Moor bath include rheumatism, arthritis, detoxification, hormonal and menstrual difficulties and skin problems including ezcema, psoriasis and acne. Full instructions as to quantity are given

on every bottle, but the basic amount of Moor used is around a fifth of a litre in each bath.

Drinking the Moor Material
Odd as it seems, the herbal constituents of the product make Moor suitable for oral use.

NEYDHARTING MOOR LIFE HERBAL DRINK
is extracted from the Moor material and is useful for a variety of disorders including rheumatic and arthritic problems, and digestive and intestinal problems including gallstones. It is ideal for use in any detoxification programme and for anyone with a sensitive digestion and tendency to liverish symptoms. It is suggested that it be taken three times daily for between four and six weeks to be most effective.

Moor products are available from: Austrian Moor Products Ltd, White Ladies, Maresfield, East Sussex TN22 2HH, UK; Nutri Centre, 7 Park Crescent, London W1N 3HE; and many health stores and pharmacies.

Israeli Dead Sea Products

Romantic Biblical and historical figures such as the Queen of Sheba, Cleopatra, King Solomon and King David are all said to have had curative bathing palaces on the Dead Sea in ancient times. The Dead Sea (really a vast inland lake) and its adjacent hot springs differ from all other known bodies of water in that the exceptionally high concentrations of mineral salts (nearly 28 per cent – four times more than sea water) make the water so dense that you cannot sink in it – it fully supports your weight. Chemical analysis of water and mud from this lowest place on the planet (it is nearly

400 metres below sea level) shows an enormous content of minerals including iodine, bromine, chloride, carbonic acid, sulphates, sodium, potassium, calcium, magnesium, lithium, strontium, hydrogen sulphide and radium.

Apart from having remarkable (and well-researched) healing effects on skin conditions such as psoriasis, the Dead Sea products that are now available have a wide range of applications for health and beauty enhancement. Any home health spa should have them in stock:

DEAD SEA MINERAL SALTS BATH

Finders, the importers of Dead Sea products into the UK, recommend that anyone with rheumatic or arthritic or general aches, pains and stiffness take a series of luke-warm baths (around 37°C or up to 40°C if you have rheumatic pain) into which a pack of the salt is dissolved – you can use up to two packs for a more powerful salt bath. You are recommended to soak for between half an hour and an hour in the water before towelling dry and applying a mineral-rich Dead Sea moisturising agent.

The main indications are for alleviation of aches and pains, whether muscular or joint, as well as for skin conditions such as eczema and psoriasis. If there are health problems of this sort three or four treatments weekly for a month are recommended.

These Dead Sea salt baths are completely safe and no side effects should be anticipated.

DERMABALANCE MUD MASK

The black mud from the Dead Sea contains over 20 minerals and trace elements, many of which are absorbed through the skin on application as a facial mask. The effect is to exfoliate (remove dead skin), to draw impurities through the skin and to increase local circulation. When used for acne the mask is said to be enhanced by the use of Dermabalance Spot Treatment, another Dead Sea product, afterwards.

The Dead Sea range of products is very large and includes scalp and general body applications for different types of skin and for many different health problems. These include baths, mud packs for the face, exfoliant creams, lotions and moisturisers for body and face, day and night creams and ointments. They are available from: Finders International Ltd, Goudhurst, Kent TN17 1JY, UK; Nutri Centre, 7 Park Crescent, London W1N 3HE; and many health stores and pharmacies.

French Clay

Clay is a most remarkable natural substance, with the power to absorb and retain toxic materials. It is used in industry on an enormous scale. This ability to draw into itself, and to hold fast to, toxic matter means that when clay is used for health or beauty, internally or externally, it has to come from very pure sites, where no pollution might have contaminated it. This is why French clay is usually mined from a depth of 60 metres or more along the banks of pristine rivers, usually in wooded areas. The sand-free clay is then sun-dried before packing.

The chemical composition of pure clay includes large quantities of silica, iron, calcium, magnesium, zinc and enzymes. The French use the clay internally for general and specific health enhancement, by stirring a teaspoon (child's dose) or two (adult dose) of the powdered material into a glass of water and drinking it – a method that has profound detoxification potential as the clay passes through the digestive tract. It is not absorbed, although minerals that it contains may be.

Among conditions that have been shown to benefit from clay are rheumatism, allergy, asthma, stomach discomfort, food poisoning, chronic inflammation of the digestive tract, headaches, and hyperactivity in children if this is related to food intolerance.

Using Clay Externally

For Beauty

For purification of the skin a face mask of green clay (for general use) or yellow clay (if there are skin problems as it contains sulphur) is ideal. Clay absorbs impurities, cleansing the skin and promoting circulation.

The mask can be prepared from the powdered clay by mixing it with water before application, or directly from a tube which is pre-mixed. Pre-mixed clay from a tube is also ideal as first aid for treating bites and stings, as well as for local application to sprains and bruises.

Green clay, the most common one, comes in the form of chunks, or bars which need to be broken up, and in this form it has to be soaked in water for about two hours before it achieves the pliable consistency needed for use. Green clay is also marketed in very fine powdered form ready for use once mixed with water, preferably pure spring water.

For Health

Clay should be applied to painful areas such as joints or muscles in a layer about 1 or 2 cm thick and immediately covered with a muslin or cotton cloth. This poultice should be left in place for not less than an hour and ideally overnight. When removed the 'used' clay should be disposed of and never reused as it will contain appreciable levels of toxins that have been drawn through the skin.

Variations on green clay include:

- white superfine clay for internal use as described above, especially for those with a sensitive digestion, and for external use as a powder for irritated skin
- yellow extra-fine clay for internal use for people with poor metabolism, and for external use as a paste for skin impurities
- red superfine clay for use internally for those who are fatigued

There are also clay-soaps made with essential oils, milk and honey – a treat for your health spa. Argiletz clay products from France are available from: Sunny Clay, PO Box 3007, London NW3 2UZ; these and other French clays can be obtained from Nutri Centre, 7 Park Crescent, London W1N 3HE.

11

Treat Your Skin, Treat Your Health

Your skin is not just the envelope which surrounds you – it is a powerful and vital organ. It might seem strange to consider it this way, but your skin is a 'second lung' through which your body eliminates a great deal of waste material – at least, it does when it is healthy. Your circulatory system carries metabolic wastes, which are produced constantly as by-products of your normal body functions, along tiny capillaries to the skin, where they pass out of you through the pores. The outer surface of the skin itself is made up of 'dead' cells which you shed all the time, but when these dead skin cells become covered with microscopically small dirt particles and oils (which you also produce yourself), the easy elimination processes of the body through the pores of the skin can be blocked or slowed, leading to blemishes, pimples and blackheads.

There are several easy ways to use water therapy to stimulate the circulation to the skin so that wastes are delivered more efficiently, and to help clear away the obstructions caused by dead skin cells and debris on the surface, so opening up the pores and enabling them to function more efficiently. Other benefits of *regularly* (it's no good just doing this now and then) treating the skin with hydrotherapy include improved tone and the mobilisation of any fatty deposits lying below the skin surface (cellulite). Clearing cellulite depends on improved circulation and drainage of the tissues, and water treatments help to achieve this splendidly.

Your overall health will also benefit when your skin is working efficiently, because your level of toxicity drops, thereby putting less strain on other organs of elimination such as the liver, kidneys, bowels and lungs. Minor problems such as chronic catarrh can improve or vanish when the skin becomes more efficient with open channels instead of blocked ones, because when the skin does its job properly there is less need for other means of removing toxins, such as excretion through the mucous membranes. Any tendency to unpleasant body odour will also improve dramatically with hydrotherapy treatments, because bacteria on the skin surface, which can cause body odour, will have less chance to operate and at the same time sweat deposits will be cleared away more efficiently.

Another spin-off of helping your skin to do its job properly is that you will have more energy available, and greater vitality, as toxic deposits are removed from the system. And of course there is the final by-product – which might actually be your main objective – firmer and clearer skin with a better colour and surface condition.

Another amazing quality that skin has is the fact that, while it is a protective envelope, it will allow some passage through itself *in both directions*. So as well as eliminating wastes, it will also allow nutrients and herbal essences in. By using special mixtures of nutrients and salts, as well as essential oils from plants, you can have a profound beneficial influence on the way your body works.

Skin Care and Treatments in Your Home Spa

There are a few methods that you should use regularly and some that you can use now and then, selectively, when you feel like it or when they are indicated by various conditions. Some work on the surface of the skin, while others work more deeply, stimulating circulating to and through the skin. Both are necessary to get the skin working efficiently. So home spa therapy includes:

- treatments aimed mainly at detoxification and skin function, at least one of which you should use regularly – daily if possible
- whole-body systemic methods, which influence circulation and general metabolism and which you should select from and apply once or twice a week
- local methods of treatment

The methods that work mainly on skin function and detoxification include:

- skin brushing
- the salt glow
- the Moor bath
- the Epsom salts bath
- the trunk pack

Those that stimulate overall circulation and improve general metabolism, as well as improving skin function, include:

- the full body pack
- sitz baths
- sauna
- stimulating showers
- aromatherapy and herbal baths

Skin Enhancement and Detoxification

Skin Brushing

Dry Method
This is best done before you wash, shower or bathe, while your skin is still dry, and it need take only a few minutes – five at most. Once you decide to start using skin brushing to improve your skin and health, you should also make up your mind that it will become a daily routine – and because it makes you feel so good (never mind looking good), very soon you will feel as lost without it as you would if you forgot to brush your teeth!

Select from a bath-mit or a loofah or a natural bristle body-brush. Make sure the room is warm and there are no draughts, because you need to have no clothes on to do this job effectively. It can be done standing, but sitting on a stool allows you to deal with the backs of the legs and other 'difficult' parts more efficiently, without having to perform contortions.

You should start brushing gently. At first expect what is called a 'red reaction', which shows that your circulation is responding to the stimulation you are giving it. The action of brushing needs to be circular, 'creeping', and firm but not irritating. The circular motion helps you avoid rubbing over one area too much – at first once or twice over any part of the skin is adequate. The 'creeping' movement has the same effect – this simply means that you gradually move from where you are circling to the next area, not by lifting the brush, but by altering the direction as you make the circular motion, so sliding gently towards the next part of the skin which is due to receive attention.

Pay particular attention to the skin on the backs of the legs and arms, as well as to your back, abdomen and chest –

where you may be more sensitive and tender. Avoid breast tissue and be very gentle on the inner thighs. If there are bits of your back that you cannot reach, use a dry towel to rub it briskly – it will not be as effective as a brush or loofah, but will be better than no friction at all.

Again it is emphasised that you should start slowly and gently. After a week or so of skin brushing the skin that was tender will be less so and you can slowly increase the pressure and vigour of your brushing.

Wet Method
To brush using the wet method, choose from the same kinds of brush (bath-mit or loofah or natural bristle skin-brush). First shower or bathe, and before drying brush the skin as described for dry brushing, but moisten the brush or loofah as well. Shower afterwards, ideally finishing with water that is around body temperature or cooler.

The Salt Glow
The salt glow is basically a skin friction using wet, coarse sea salt or Epsom salts. It is particularly beneficial for people who have difficulty sweating or who have poor circulation to their hands or feet and is also useful for people prone to rheumatic aches and pains. The salt glow is best done *to* you, and with self-treatment it is necessary to accept that bits of your body are not going to be reached – you can't effectively friction *all* of your back yourself! Unlike skin brushing, which is suggested as a daily routine, the salt glow is a now-and-then thing – perhaps once a week at most if you have difficulty sweating and once a month or so for general detoxification purposes.

MATERIALS
You will need a bowl and at least half a pound of coarse salt
or Epsom salts.

METHOD
Sit on a stool in the bath or shower and add water to the
salt in the bowl to moisten it – just enough to make the salt
grains stick together. Take a small amount into each hand (a
tablespoonful approximately) and starting with one foot
work the salt onto the skin as you come up the leg using up
and down and circular motions. Try to friction firmly, even
vigorously, on skin that is usually exposed, such as on the
legs, so that all the skin gets some rubbing and some salt.
Work up each leg and then do each arm. Next work the salt
onto the skin around your back without straining yourself
(if a partner is there they could usefully do this for you).
Then apply the salt (rubbing firmly but not irritatingly) to
the abdomen and chest and up to the neck, avoiding breast
tissue.

After the salt rub you need to shower, ideally using a hand
shower and warm water to cleanse the surface of the skin.
As the water is playing on each area, use your free hand to
rub the salt and water off the skin, giving the area a bit more
friction as you do so. Dry with a vigorous towelling down
and go to bed – make sure the bed and the room are warm.
You should sleep very well. You may perspire heavily the first
few times you use the salt glow. As your skin becomes more
efficient, so will this heavy perspiration lessen as time passes.
Have water by the bed in case you get thirsty.

The Moor Bath
When you use a peat-like substance called Moor in a bath
you are adding the concentrated natural product of hundreds

of thousands of years of compression of the organic materials from decaying mosses, leaves and roots. The resulting 'soup' contains rich supplies of silica, sulphur, iron, resins and many minerals and harmless acids. Many of these ingredients help to neutralise harmful toxins on and under the skin, and since many of the micro-elements in Moor can be absorbed through the skin, it can also influence your general health. There are particular benefits to skin and rheumatic problems, although medical research has also shown that Moor baths can help blood pressure problems, circulatory difficulties and in restoring balance when there are sugar disturbances.

MATERIALS
Liquid Moor peat from pharmacies, specialist beauty suppliers or health stores.

METHOD
The very best way of using Moor is to apply it as a paste to the body surface as a whole, but while this can be done effectively at health spas it is not a practical proposition in the home. By using liquid Moor you can enjoy the health benefits of Moor at home. All you need do is pour the liquid (amounts will be indicated on the container) into a hot bath and soak for between 20 and 30 minutes. You should shower well afterwards and retire to a warm bed. As with the salt glow you might expect to perspire more than usual that night and to sleep very well indeed. Have water by your bed to drink in order to make up the liquid lost through sweating, and be prepared to change your sheets next morning.

How often you use this method depends on your needs. If you are rheumatic and have an acidic tendency then a Moor bath every week would be a good idea. If you just want to experience Moor and give your skin a boost from its wonderful ingredients, then once or twice a month is adequate.

For more on the therapeutic and beauty uses of Moor, mud and clay, see chapter 10.

The Epsom Salts Bath and Flotation Tanks

There are few more effective ways of stimulating skin function than an Epsom salts bath. It dramatically increases elimination through the skin and, as in the case of the Moor bath, is ideal if there is any tendency towards acidity, rheumatic problems, or if there is a need to detoxify (and this applies to almost everyone nowadays).

CONTRA-INDICATIONS
Anyone with a serious cardiac condition, or diabetes, or who has a skin condition that is 'open' or weeping should not use this method.

MATERIALS
Epsom salts (from any good pharmacy), sea salt, iodine.

METHOD
Into a comfortably hot bath place one pound of commercial Epsom salts plus a quarter to half a pound of sea salt and a dessertspoonful of iodine (get the clear variety to avoid staining the bath). This combination of salts and iodine approximates the constituents of the sea. Stay in the bath, just lying there as it is quite impossible to wash in this salt mixture, for not less than 10 minutes and not more than 20. Top up with hot water if you stay in beyond 10 minutes to keep the water feeling hot. When you get out do not shower – just towel yourself dry and get into a pre-warmed bed.

Once again, as with the peat bath and the salt glow, you should expect to sweat heavily, and to sleep even more heavily. Have water by the bed as you may need to top up the lost liquid. In the morning take a shower and apply a moisturiser to the skin as a whole.

It is not recommended that you take an Epsom salts bath more than once a week, and once a month is probably the ideal for general detoxification purposes and stimulation of skin function.

Simulated Flotation Tank

A novel way of achieving deep relaxation involves the so-called flotation tank, in which you are suspended in very buoyant water inside a light-proof tank. The absence of any stimuli has a profoundly calming effect, although some people find the experience claustrophobic.

The method was first developed during the Second World War by Dr John Lilly, who researched the effects of sensory deprivation and found that floating in water without effort, if the eyes are masked from light and the temperature of the water is neither hot nor cold, produces a profoundly relaxing effect. Anxiety, depression, fatigue and tension, as well as a wide range of painful conditions and even high blood pressure, all responded positively to the method, which evolved into the flotation tank in which you simply float in water saturated with Epsom salts (rather like being in the Dead Sea).

You can approximate the benefits without danger of claustrophobia at home by running an Epsom salts bath with sea salt (as above) at neutral (body heat) temperature, since this comes very close to the consistency and buoyancy of a flotation tank. Use an eye mask and have some pleasant music in the background, and just lie there for 20 minutes or so, topping up the water with hot when it cools at all.

The Trunk Pack

This is a modification of the full-body wet-sheet pack (see next page and Chapter 12), but is less difficult to apply and also less demanding on your energy – the wet-sheet pack can leave you feeling a bit limp for a day or so at first. Its objective is to stimulate elimination through the skin but also to influence circulation through the pelvic and abdominal areas.

MATERIALS
A large bath towel or a strip of blanket; a strip of cotton material; safety pins; a blanket.

METHOD
Fold a thick towel in two or three or have available a piece of blanket, wide enough to cover the area from your armpit to your navel and long enough to go right around you with some overlap. Onto this place one thickness of damp, well-wrung-out cotton material which is at least an inch less wide than the covering material and which can wrap around you once without overlap. Place these on a bed and lie on the material, wrapping it over to cover the entire area between your navel and your armpits. Quickly fold and safety-pin it, or have someone do this for you. Cover yourself with a blanket and rest.

The cold, damp cotton should warm very rapidly if it is well wrapped with no damp edges protruding, not too wet (it needs to have been well wrung out) and firmly pinned. If it fails to warm within five minutes take it off, briskly friction the skin and abandon the treatment for that day. Otherwise keep the pack on for not less than an hour and ideally for three to four hours so that it is virtually dry by the time it is taken off. The best way is to sleep with it on, but it can be done during the day if you can stay resting. The cotton must be well washed before reusing as it absorbs a lot of acidic wastes from the skin.

Use this treatment once or twice a month as an alternative to the more aggressive methods, such as the Epsom salts bath and the salt glow, if you find these too difficult.

Whole-Body Water Treatments

The Full-Body Wet-Sheet Pack
The description of this treatment is in chapter 12. Abbreviated comments are given here.

After an initial cool stage, which should last no more than five minutes, there is a neutral stage, when the pack is the same temperature as the body, which produces a profound calming effect if you are agitated, anxious or nervous. This stage may last for half an hour or more depending upon how quickly your body heat warms the material containing the water, and if the effect you are looking for is relaxation then this is the time to get yourself unwrapped (which is hard without help, so have someone close by to release you).

If you are also interested in detoxification you need to, let the pack go on working through the next two stages: a hot stage, which is most useful for pain problems such as sinus congestion or bowel discomfort (especially if constipated), and which lasts for anything from half an hour to an hour; and the sweating stage, in which sweating becomes profuse while detoxification is taking place, and which can last for up to an hour. At this stage have a cold wet towel placed on your forehead and if necessary drink something (through a straw because your hands are wrapped in the pack with you).

For a full description of the method of application of the full-body wet-sheet pack, and the materials you'll need, see chapter 12, pages 112–15.

Sitz Baths

The full description of this method is in chapter 12, pages 118–20, in the section on Partial Alternate Bathing.

Sauna

Unless you are lucky enough to have a sauna at home this needs to be a treat you give yourself when you go along to a local health club or sauna bath.

In the wood-lined room of the traditional Scandinavian sauna you are exposed to a dry-heat bath which induces a great deal of perspiration. The effects are profound, and generally include a great deal of tension release and relaxation, along with the enormous elimination produced via the sweating.

The benefits to circulation are well researched and proven, and anyone with a skin problem such as acne can be sure there will be an improvement after the skin has opened in the dry heat. Muscular and joint aches and stiffness are relieved and breathing problems also benefit. Circulation is even further enhanced if the skin is stimulated during the sauna. And you don't have to use birch twigs in the way the Finnish people do – you can just briskly rub your skin with a loofah or bath-mit every now and then while sitting in the sauna.

If you are not used to sauna you should stick to a 20-minute introduction followed by a tepid shower (or a cold one – remember the Finns dive into snow after theirs!) and a full body massage. One sauna a month is a wonderful aid to regular detoxification and skin cleansing – you can do it more often if you like, but probably not more than once a week.

RECOMMENDED ROUTINE
Take a short warm shower followed by 10 to 15 minutes in
the sauna, then a 30-second cool or cold plunge (many
saunas have plunge baths available for this purpose) or
shower. A few minutes rest in the warm room is a good idea
at this time. Have another 10 to 15 minutes in the sauna once
you are used to the process, followed again by a cool shower
or plunge, and a rest. A massage rounds out a super
indulgence which will do wonders for you and your skin.

When you are in the sauna you will notice benches, some
of which are nearer the ceiling than others, and clearly these
are the hottest ones. By adapting to the lower bench first and
only moving to the higher ones later you let your body
acclimatise to what is a novel experience for most of us.

Don't eat for an hour before or an hour after a sauna, but
replenish with liquid whenever you feel the need. Take
medical advice before using a sauna if you have any serious
medical condition, especially diabetes or a heart condition.

Stimulating Showers
Modern shower heads are remarkably adaptable and capable
of producing a wide variety of jets, ranging from a blast to
a delicate spray or even an alternating pulsating series of jets.
For water therapy in the shower you have a vast range of
choices and these include:

- *varying the temperature* from hot (relaxing) to tepid (very
  relaxing) to cool or even cold (stimulating and
  energising)
- *varying the timing* – by keeping the period of heat or
  cold longer or shorter you can achieve different effects
- *varying the amount of pressure* being delivered to the skin
  by the pressurised shower head

- *using the knowledge of reflex areas* to achieve effects in different areas of the body (see pages 53–4)

If you can achieve alternation of temperature quickly, as well as alternation of pressure of water, you have a powerful tool for home hydrotherapy. The benefits include

- a tonic effect for the circulation (and therefore the skin), which can be general or local
- relaxation or stimulation depending on the choices made of the variables
- easing of aches and stiffness
- rapid cleansing of the skin and pores

Let's look at some of the choices you have.

A Hot Shower

Heat relaxes but also enervates or tires you, so do not have a hot shower for a long period (never longer than five minutes) and remember that heat should always be followed by a cool or cold (or at the very least tepid) application of water if you want to help circulation and skin tone. You will clean the skin more effectively with a hot than a cold shower, so use the opportunity to brush vigorously or use a scrub material or wash with pH balanced soap.

If you want to have the hot shower playing onto a stiff or aching area, say your back or a knee, let this be accompanied by placing a cool damp towel on your head while the heat is building in the local area being treated.

A Cold Shower

The effect of cold water is to constrict and contract whatever it is in touch with, so a very brief cold shower, either to finish after a hot one or on its own, will have an extremely stimulating effect and will actually leave you glowing with inner warmth afterwards, especially if you dry yourself briskly. A minute or two is enough for this effect, and remember that it leads to fewer infections (see chapter 6).

The Neutral Shower

Just like the neutral bath or the second stage of the full sheet pack, a neutral shower (at body heat, so that it feels neither hot nor cold) will have a calming, balancing effect. You can stay in it for as long as you like, even getting a stool into the shower space and sitting there for 10 or 15 minutes if this allows you to become really relaxed.

Alternating Showers

Using alternating hot and cold water allows you to clear the skin, relax the muscles and stimulate the circulation – an amazing series of achievements for just three or four minutes of effort. Start warm and get hotter, taking around one to two minutes to get really hot, then change quickly to a cold shower for 15 seconds, and then go back to hot and then cold, and so on. Or you can stop after one or two alternations if you feel you have done enough for your circulation for one day!

You will feel marvellous and there are no contra-indications. The degree of coldness and hotness you use is up to you and your tolerance. Slowly get yourself to the point where you can not only stand a big contrast (not just going from warm to cool), but actually start to enjoy the thrill of the contrast from hot to cold – and back again.

You can also use the pressure feature of the shower head

to play on areas of the body where you feel you need to improve circulation or influence reflex areas.

Aromatherapy and Other Beauty Baths

Some of the baths described below are aimed at stress reduction, since anyone who is feeling stressed and anxious is clearly not operating at their optimum, and this will influence the way you look and feel. So for energy and well-being, as well as for glowing good looks, pay attention to anti-stress measures. Various strategies such as relaxation, sound nutrition and exercise, are necessary to combat stress, and aromatherapy baths are an enjoyable addition to them. They are only contra-indicated for people with skins that are sensitive or allergic to whatever is being used in the bath.

Anti-stress Aromatherapy Bath

Into a hot bath place the following cocktail of Mediterranean oils

10 drops each of rosemary and aniseed oils
5 drops each of basil and pine oils
3 drops each of eucalyptus and cypress oils

OR

10 drops each of bergamot and sandalwood oils
5 drops each of cinnamon and sage oils
3 drops each of clove and coriander oils

Use a sponge to gently work the oils into your skin – no soap is used in a bath such as this. The effect of a bath lasting 10 to 20 minutes in either of these combinations will be a profound feeling of refreshment and relaxation. Pat dry without friction, and rest afterwards.

Calming Herbal Bath

A herbal bath, which uses leaves and flowers instead of oils to calm and soothe, is ideal for bedtime and when nerves are really on edge or when insomnia is a problem. From a herbal supplier or wholefood shop obtain at least five of the following – the more the better.

¼ oz *each* of marigold flowers and yarrow flower heads
½ oz *each* of orange leaves, lemon leaves, chamomile flowers, peppermint leaves, linden flowers, lemon verbena leaves, wild poppy petals
6 oz oat bran
2.5 l mineral water

Place the water and bran into a large saucepan, bring to the boil and allow to simmer for 3 or 4 minutes, during which time add as many of the herbal ingredients as you have been able to obtain. Remove from the heat and let it cool for 10–15 minutes. Strain the essence of the oatmeal and herbs and put this liquid into a hot bath which you will have run while the mixture was cooling.

What is left behind in the saucepan when you have strained the liquid is placed in cotton or muslin or cheesecloth material and tied firmly with string to make a 'sponge' for the bath. Soak for 15 minutes using the sponge to rub your skin gently – no soap is used. Go to bed after patting yourself dry, and sleep deeply.

Luxury Milk and Honey Bath

For this luxurious bath you require the following

2 oz (50g) liquid honey (acacia or heather are ideal)
2 l cows milk
10 drops each of the following essential oils – lemon,
clove and cinnamon
5 drops of sandalwood essential oil

Dissolve the honey in hot milk, then run a hot bath into which all the ingredients are placed early. Soak for as long as you like (think of Cleopatra – she couldn't have done better) and use a natural sponge to gently rub the essences into your skin – don't bother with soap. Pat dry and sleep like a queen.

Toning Herbal Bath

To boost energy and breathing function, try this special herbal bath. Try to obtain at least five of the plant ingredients.

¼ oz each of bay leaves, eucalyptus leaves, peppermint
leaves, juniper leaves, pine needles, rosemary leaves,
thyme leaves, marjoram leaves
2 oz rice flour
2.5 l spring water

Place the water into a large saucepan and, before starting to heat it, add the rice flour. It requires a bit of effort to mix the flour with the water, so use a fork or whisk to get it well mixed, then place it on the heat and bring to the boil. You need to stir it frequently to keep the rice flour in suspension while it is heating. When it is boiling, add the herbs and remove from the heat, allowing it to cool for at least 15 minutes during which time run a hot bath. Strain the liquid into the bath and soak for 10 to 15 minutes, using a cloth or sponge to rub the skin firmly (the rice flour in the water will act as a mild abrasive 'scrub').

You should feel invigorated and energised after the bath.

Skin Tonic Herbal Bath

Obtain at least five of the flowers or herbs, fresh or dry.

¼ oz each of marigold flowers, chamomile flowers, rose flowers, rosemary leaves, sage leaves
1 oz lavender flowers
6 oz wheat bran
3 oz oatmeal (fine)
2.5 l spring water

Put the water, bran and oatmeal in a large saucepan and bring to the boil, stirring periodically. When it is boiling, add the flowers and herbs and remove from the heat for 15 minutes while you run a hot bath. Strain the liquid into the bath and put the solid material left over into a muslin or cotton or cheesecloth bag to use as a sponge. During the bath rub your skin with the bag, and afterwards pat dry and go to bed. You should perspire freely and your skin should feel smoother and softer.

Simple Detox Bath

For a simple Epsom salt bath to encourage relaxation, easing of stiffness or aches and for strong detoxification, dissolve between 2 and 4 lb in the hot water and soak in this for 20 minutes. Briskly rub dry and get into warm bed. Expect to perspire profusely.

Single Oil Baths

For essential oil baths to achieve specific effects, such as chamomile for relaxation and pain relief, use a few drops of the oil in the bath and soak for up to half an hour. See chapter 9 on aromatic oils for their properties and indications and choose accordingly.

Oatmeal Bath

For an oatmeal bath, ideal for any skin irritations, take 1 lb uncooked oatmeal and place it in a gauze bag which should be held under the hot tap as it runs, thereby releasing the ingredients which are soothing to the skin. Float the bag in the bath while soaking in it and use it as a sponge to gently pat areas of irritation. The temperature of the bath should be around 96°F or 36°C. Stay in the bath for at least 20 minutes. Pat dry afterwards, without rubbing.

Romantic Aromatherapy or Herbal Bath

Essential oils and aromatic herbs can set the scene for romance and the following suggestions give you a starting point. There are many other possibilities, so try your own combinations.

OILS
Add to a bath the following (ideally when bath is half full and still running)

    3 to 5 drops of patchouli
    3 drops of lavender
    2 drops of rose

OR

3 to 5 drops of ylang ylang
3 drops of vetiver
3 drops of geranium

PLANT PETALS
Add three or four of the following to a saucepan of boiling
water, remove from the heat immediately and allow to cool
for 15 minutes before adding the strained essence to the bath:

½ oz each of petals of rose, carnation, lily, honeysuckle
(these can be used fresh), lavender, clover and
geranium leaves (these are best used dried)

To round off the romantic bath, massage with a mixture of
either of the following, in carrier oil:

2 drops patchouli
2 drops lavender
2 drops sandalwood

OR

2 drops ylang ylang
2 drops basil
2 drops sandalwood

Energy-boosting Herbal Baths
Choose from one of the following combinations:

lavender
peppermint
lemon verbena

comfrey leaf or root

OR

   sage
   patchouli leaf
   thyme
   bay (or eucalyptus)
   sandalwood chips

OR

   bay
   rosemary
   rose
   chamomile
   peppermint

Take half an ounce of each ingredient and place in a large saucepan with 2 to 3 litres of water. Bring to the boil and allow to simmer for 15 minutes. Place the strained liquid in a warm or hot bath and soak for 20 minutes.

Relaxing Herbal Baths

   1 oz chamomile
   ½ oz each of linden flowers, violet leaves, hops or comfrey

Place the herbs in a saucepan with 3 litres of water and bring to the boil. Let this simmer for 15 minutes. Strain and place the liquid in a hot bath and soak for at least 20 minutes.

Herbal Bath for Dry Skin
Half a ounce of at least four of the following:

chamomile, rose petals, rosemary, violets (leaf or flower or both), comfrey leaf or comfrey root or both, acacia flowers

Place in saucepan with 2.5 to 3 litres of water, bring to the boil and allow to simmer for 15 minutes. Strain and place the fluid in a bath. Soak and pat dry when finished.

Herbal Bath for Oily Skin
Half an ounce each of at least four of the following:

witch hazel bark, lemon peel, raspberry leaf, lemon grass, peppermint, orange flowers or peel, chamomile

Place in saucepan with 2.5 to 3 litres of water, bring to the boil and allow to simmer for 15 minutes. Strain and place the fluid in a bath. Soak and pat dry when finished.

Local Treatments for Skin Care

The Face Sauna
You can buy inexpensive equipment which will allow steam to be brought to your face for cosmetic purposes, although far cheaper is the use of a bowl and a towel or umbrella. For cleansing the pores deeply as well as toning and softening the skin, the home face sauna is a super-efficient method.
Add the use of essential oils or herbs for extra benefits.

Herbs

GENERAL CLEANSING FACE SAUNA
Use at least four of the following herbs:

> half an ounce each of rose petals, lavender, chamomile
> flowers, elder blossom, acacia, mint, sage, chickweed,
> comfrey leaf and/or root, raspberry leaf, strawberry
> leaf, slippery elm bark

Add the herbs to 2 litres of water in a saucepan. Bring this
to the boil and allow to simmer for two to three minutes.
Remove from the heat and allow to cool for a minute or so,
and then place a towel over your entire head to drape over
your face and the bowl so that your face (eyes closed) is in
direct touch with the rising herb-laden steam. Stay in the
steam for at least five and ideally ten minutes and then splash
the face with cold water and pat dry.

FOR NORMAL AND DRY SKINS
Use the same method as for the previous face sauna, but this
time use an ounce each of peppermint and chamomile and
2 ounces of lemongrass.

FOR OILY SKIN
As above, but this time use an ounce each of basil, comfrey
root and rosemary.

Essential Oils

FOR DRY, NORMAL AND MATURE SKINS
Bring a litre of water to the boil and allow it to cool for two
minutes. Pour it into a bowl and add four drops each of

geranium and lavender oil and two drops of patchouli. Cover your entire head and the bowl with a towel and let the vapours treat your skin for five minutes or so.

FOR OILY SKIN
As above, but this time add four drops each of lemon, cypress and juniper oils.

NOTE
Always use a skin toner or freshener after steaming and, if there is a tendency to dryness, a natural moisturiser as well.

See chapter 10 on the uses of mud, Moor and clay for other local treatments of the skin.

12

Water Therapy for General Health and Symptom Control

The range of hydrotherapy methods for you to use at home represents only a small part of what might be available at a modern European or American hydrotherapy clinic or spa. This is because the methods outlined in this book have been selected above all for safety, for relative ease of application, and also for their proven effectiveness. Most act in a general way – they are not specific treatments, but methods which by helping circulation, detoxification and general relaxation will support the constant effort of the body to heal itself and to become more efficient and effective. This chapter describes the most effective treatments for home use, all of which have considerable benefits for general health.

Heating Compress
This is called a cold compress in Europe. It is a simple but effective method involving a piece of cold, wet material (cotton is best), *well* wrung out in cold water and then applied to an area which is immediately covered in a way that insulates it and allows your body heat to warm the cold material. Plastic is also often used to prevent the damp from spreading and to further insulate the material.

The effect is for a reflex stimulus to take place when the cold material first touches the skin, leading to a flushing away from the tissues of 'old' blood and a return to them of fresh, oxygenated blood. As the compress slowly warms there is a deeply relaxing effect and a reduction of pain.

This is an ideal method for self-treatment or first aid for any of the following:

- painful joints
- mastitis
- sore throat (compress on the throat from ear to ear and supported over the top of the head)
- backache (ideally the compress should cover the abdomen and the back)
- sore tight chest from bronchitis

MATERIALS

- A single or double piece of cotton sheeting large enough to cover the area to be treated (double for people with good circulation and vitality, single for people with only moderate circulation and vitality)
- One thickness of woollen or flannel material (towelling will do but is not as effective) *larger* than the cotton material so that it can cover it completely with no edges protruding
- Plastic material of the same size as the woollen material
- Safety pins
- Cold water

METHOD

Ring out the cotton material in cold water so that it is damp but not dripping wet. Place this over the painful area and immediately cover it with the woollen or flannel material, and also the plastic material if used, and pin the covering snugly in place. The compress should be firm enough to ensure that no air can get in to cool it, but not so tight as to impede circulation. The cold material should rapidly warm and feel comfortable, and after several hours it should be virtually dry.

Wash the material before reusing it as it will absorb acid wastes from the body.

Use a warming compress up to four times daily with at least an hour between applications if it is found to be helpful for any of the conditions listed above. Ideally leave it on overnight.

CAUTION
If for any reason the compress is still cold after 20 minutes (the compress may be too wet or too loose, or the vitality may not be adequate to the task of warming it), then remove it and give the area a brisk rub with a towel.

Fomentations
The application of damp heat to an area leads to an increased circulation to that region, followed by increased metabolic activity involving the whole body, sweating, tissue relaxation and reduction in pain or spasm.

Fomentations are useful for

- pain and congestion, especially involving muscle spasm and tension
- lumbago and neuralgia between the ribs
- dysmenorrhoea (painful periods)
- kidney stones (renal colic)

CONTRA-INDICATIONS
Do not use fomentations in all cases of cancer, heart disease, diabetes mellitus, circulatory problems of the legs, haemorrhage, or sensitive skin.

MATERIALS

- Sheet
- Blanket
- Towels
- Very hot water
- Woollen material for fomentation (a towel will do but is less efficient)
- Bowl with hot water (and mustard if you want it to be super-efficient)
- Bowl with cold water or access to cold water tap
- Hot water bottle (for Method 2)

METHOD 1

This treatment is impossible to do for yourself so someone has to help with the applications.

Sit in an upright chair with your feet in a bowl of bearably hot water (104°F or 40°C) in which two or three teaspoonsful of mustard powder have been dissolved. Uncover the area to be treated and have the sheet and blanket handy to cover this and as much of the body as possible once the fomentation has been applied. Lightly wring out the woollen or towelling fomentation material in very hot water (the more water retained the more effective the fomentation) and place this immediately between several layers of dry, larger towels. Apply the insulated hot towels to the painful area and cover immediately with the sheet and blanket. If the fomentation is too hot for comfort, remove it for a few seconds, dry the skin, and then replace it.

Change to a new fomentation application every five minutes, but between each application place a cold wet towel on the area for a few (5 to 10) seconds. After the second fomentation application, or when sweating begins, apply a cold towel to the forehead. Repeat the applications of hot fomentations a total of three or four times. After the last fomentation is removed use a damp, cold towel to friction the area, and the body as a whole, briskly (except if you are treating dysmenorrhoea) and then rest in a warm and comfortable position for half an hour to an hour.

This treatment can be done daily if helpful, but the skin should be protected by vaseline or something similar if it is repeated frequently.

The heat of fomentations promotes sweating and elimination of toxic wastes. It also relaxes local spasm, thus reducing pain.

METHOD 2
Lie down on an open sheet and blanket with a hot water bottle by your feet. The material to be used for the fomentation should be wrung out in very hot water, placed between the insulating towels and applied to the area being treated. Cover with the sheet and blanket and leave for four to five minutes. Then remove it and apply a cold compress to the head while preparing the next fomentation. Apply three fomentations.

Finish off (after the last fomentation has been removed) with a friction of your whole body using a mitten or towel. Wrap yourself in the sheet and blanket and rest for at least half an hour.

Neutral Bath
By placing yourself in a neutral bath in which your body temperature is the same as that of the water, a profoundly relaxing influence on the nervous system occurs. This was the main method of calming violent and disturbed patients in mental asylums before tranquillisers appeared!

A neutral bath is useful in all cases of anxiety, for feelings of being stressed and for relieving chronic pain and insomnia. It is ideal for reducing excessive fluid if retention is a problem, and it is a general tonic for the heart.

CONTRA-INDICATIONS
Do not use with skin conditions which react badly to water, or if there is serious cardiac disease. In the latter case it may help, but get professional advice first.

MATERIALS
A bathtub, water and a bath thermometer.

METHOD
Run a bath as full as possible and with the water as close to 97°F (36.1°C) as possible, and certainly not exceeding that level. The bath has its effect by being as close to body temperature as you can achieve. Immersion in water at this neutral temperature has a profoundly relaxing, sedating effect and a calming influence on nervous system activity.

Get into the bath so that the water covers your shoulders, and support the back of your head on a towel or sponge. The thermometer should be in the bath so that you can make sure that the temperature does not drop below 92°F (33.3°C). The water can be topped up periodically, *but must not exceed the 97°F/36.1°C limit*. The duration of the bath should be anything from 30 minutes to four hours – the longer the better for maximum relaxation.

After the bath pat dry quickly and get into bed for at least an hour.

Full Sheet Pack
The way a wet-sheet pack works depends on how you use it. The full sheet pack is remarkable in that it passes through

four distinct stages of activity, each of which has different effects on the person receiving it and is therefore useful for treating different conditions. The four stages are:

1 An initial cooling stage useful for feelings of general weakness or if there is a fever. This stage lasts no more than five minutes.
2 A neutral stage, when the pack is the same temperature as the body, which has the same effects as a neutral bath, and is particularly helpful for agitation, anxiety and nervousness. This stage may last for half an hour or more depending upon how quickly your body heat warms the wet material.
3 A hot stage, which helps in a number of health conditions but is most useful for pain problems such as sinus congestion, bowel discomfort (especially if constipated) or conditions such as colitis.
4 A stage when sweating becomes profuse, which is used for general detoxification and to assist the elimination of the residues of drugs, including tobacco. It can also be used during some infections to hasten the fever process, but only under supervision.

CONTRA-INDICATIONS
Avoid stages three and four if you are very anaemic or very weak or debilitated. Being wrapped, mummy-like, can be claustrophobic, so there should always be someone on hand to help with removal of the pack in case this happens or if you feel unwell. Do not use this treatment if you have a skin condition that is made worse by water. Anyone with diabetes should take advice before using a wet-sheet pack.

MATERIALS

- Two cotton sheets
- Two wool blankets
- Towels
- A pillow
- A hot water bottle
- A hand towel

METHOD

This treatment is impossible to do for yourself, so have someone on hand to help you with the application.

Place a blanket on the bed, open fully. Have a warm shower, and on emerging from this without drying yourself get your helper to wrap you in a cold wet sheet, which should have been well wrung out in water at between 60 and 70°F (15–21°C). The younger and more vital the person receiving the pack, the more water can be left in the sheet, but it should never be dripping wet when applied.

Working swiftly, the damp cold sheet should be wrapped from under your armpits so that it fits snugly to your body right down to the ankles, and should be immediately covered by a second, dry sheet before you lie down on the blanket, which should then be wrapped around you from neck to feet with no sheet visible (thus avoiding contact with the air, which would keep it cool). The second blanket should be placed over the first one and tucked around you snugly. Use towels and/or a neck pillow to insulate areas such as the neck where the blanket may not efficiently be enclosing the pack. Place a hot water bottle near the feet. *Speed of operation is essential* as chilling will occur if the work is done slowly. When the third and fourth stages are reached (the pack feels hot and you start to sweat), a cold compress to the forehead is a good idea, as would be the offer of sips of water if you feel thirsty

– sweating can be profuse in stage four so water replenishment is necessary.

The pack can be discontinued at or after any of the four stages as appropriate. For full benefit it should run its course, which takes up to three hours or more depending on your vitality, that is, how quickly you heat the sheet. If at any time after the first few minutes the pack is uncomfortably cold the treatment should be stopped and a brisk friction applied to the whole body surface using a mitten or dry towel to stimulate circulation. The failure of the sheet to warm up would indicate either that the sheet was too wet or the water too cold, or that the insulation was inadequately applied.

Ice-Pack

Ice decongests the tissues it is passing over as it melts because of the amazing amount of heat it has to absorb to turn from solid into liquid. Ice treatment is helpful for

- all sprains and injuries
- bursitis and other joint swellings or inflammations
- (unless cold aggravates the pain)
- toothache
- headache
- haemorrhoids
- bites

CONTRA-INDICATIONS
Do not use abdominal application during acute bladder problems, over the chest with acute asthma or if any health condition is aggravated by cold.

MATERIALS

- A piece of flannel or wool material large enough to cover the area to be treated
- Towels
- Ice
- Safety pins
- Plastic
- Bandage

METHOD

Place crushed ice to form a thickness of an inch or so onto a towel, then fold and pin the towel to contain the ice. Place the wool or flannel material onto the site of the pain and put the ice-pack onto this. Cover the pack with plastic and use the bandage to hold the whole thing in place. Protect clothing and bedding with additional plastic and towels.

Leave the pack in place for up to half an hour, and repeat after an hour if helpful.

Ice Massage

Use either ice (messy as it melts) or something metallic that has been in a freezer. For example, you can empty a soft-drink can of its previous contents, fill it with water and freeze it. Seal the hole, and use the can to roll over the painful area to chill it, ensuring that the skin does not frost or become irritated. Several minutes of slowly moving iced metal over a joint or other painful area will relieve a good deal of pain. If at the same time gentle stretching or painless movement can be introduced, the benefits are enhanced.

Alternatively, try a cold spray such as those used on injuries to reactivate fallen warriors on the sports-field. Take care with these sprays as they can blanch and damage the skin, although if used in slow sweeps they are very useful.

Ice massage is ideal for acute problems or for regular symptomatic relief of chronic joint problems.

Steam Inhalation

Steam penetrates and can be used to reach areas unavailable to any other method, on its own or as a carrier of essential oils or herbal essences. Steam inhalation is helpful for a painful, tight chest during respiratory infections, for sore throats, and for sinus problems.

For skin care a face sauna or steam-bath opens the pores and allows for a number of other helpful substances to be absorbed. Try adding four drops of rosemary, camomile or peppermint to a bowl of steaming water. Follow this with a cold splash and whatever additional skin care you wish to use.

CONTRA-INDICATIONS

Do not use steam inhalation if there is cardiac asthma or a serious heart condition, or if you are too frail to cope with the heat of steam.

MATERIALS

- Kettle and hot water
- Bowl
- Sheet
- Umbrella, towel or sheet
- Roll of newspaper (optional)
- Essential oils such as eucalyptus or wintergreen, or leaves such as mint (aromatic herbs are optional)

METHOD
Bring the kettle to the boil and place it safely so that you can be seated close by, covered by a 'tent' made out of the umbrella and draped sheet which also encloses the steaming kettle. A few drops of the oil or the leaves of plants can be placed in the kettle and the roll of paper placed over the spout to direct the steam towards your face (this is not essential). Breathe the steam slowly and deeply, avoiding any scalding of the skin, which could occur if you are too close to the spout. Take care not to upset the kettle. Periodically use a cold damp towel to cool your face and forehead. Thirty minutes of steam inhalation, three times daily, helps relieve congestion.

METHOD 2
Add boiling water and a few drops of essential oil to a bowl. Cover your entire head with a towel and place your face over the steam from the bowl – not too close or you'll irritate your skin – and keep your eyes closed. Breathe slowly and deeply for up to 15 minutes or until the steam ceases rising.

Partial Alternate Bathing
By alternating hot and cold water in different ways it is possible to have profound effects on circulation, and through the circulation to influence many aspects of your health, including feeling more energetic and having a clearer complexion. Alternate bathing is useful for all conditions that involve congestion and inflammation, locally or generally, and for an overall tonic effect. Alternating sitz baths are ideal for varicose veins and haemorrhoids.

CONTRA-INDICATIONS
Alternate bathing should not be used if there is

haemorrhage, colic and spasm, acute or serious chronic heart disease, or acute bladder and kidney infections.

MATERIALS

You will need containers suitable for holding hot and cold water. If the part to be immersed is the whole pelvic area, then large plastic or other tubs (an old-fashioned hip bath is best) are required, along with a smaller container for immersion of the feet at the same time. You also need a bath thermometer, hot and cold water, and for some treatments you might want special ingredients, such as mustard.

METHOD

If a local area such as the arm, wrist or ankle is receiving treatment, then that part should be alternately immersed in hot and cold water following the timings given below for alternating sitz baths. For local immersion treatment ice cubes can be placed in the cold water for greater contrast.

If the area is unsuitable for treatment by immersion (a shoulder or a knee could be awkward), then application to those regions of hot and cold temperatures is possible by using towels soaked and lightly wrung out in water of the appropriate temperature, again following the same time scales as for sitz baths, given below.

Sitz Baths

These are the immersion of the pelvic area (buttocks and hips up to the navel) in water of one temperature, with feet in water of the same or a contrasting temperature. The sequence to follow in alternating pelvic bathing in sitz baths is:

- 1–3 minutes seated in hot water (106–110°F or 41–43°C)
- 15–30 seconds in cold (around 60°F/15°C)
- 1–3 minutes hot
- 15 seconds cold

During the hip immersions the feet should *if possible* be in water of a contrasting temperature, so when the hips are in hot water, the feet should be in cold, and vice versa. If this is hard to organise, the alternating hip immersions alone should be used.

Simple Bathing
These are full or partial baths where no alternation of temperatures occurs.

Mustard Bath
This is recommended in the early stages of a developing headache.

One teaspoonful of powdered mustard is added to two gallons of hot water in a bowl large enough for both feet to rest in. A similar bowl, also containing hot mustard water, rests on the knees, and the hands and forearms are placed in it. Put a cool, damp cloth on the forehead. After 20 minutes wash the hands and feet thoroughly and rest.

Hot Sitz Bath
A hot sitz bath, with no alternation of hot and cold, but simply pelvic immersion in hot water, is of proven value in helping speed the healing of painful anal fissures, as well as haemorrhoids, dysmenorrhoea, prostate and bladder

inflammation, pelvic inflammatory disease and atonic constipation.

CONTRA-INDICATIONS
Hot sitz baths should not be used by anyone with a diabetic condition.

MATERIALS
As for alternate bathing, although a regular bath tub may be used.

METHOD
If a hip bath is available, then sit in it in hot water (106–110°F or 41–43°C) with the feet in water a few degrees hotter. If a regular bath is used, sit in it in hot water up to the navel, knees bent so that they are out of the water, and feet immersed. Apply a cold towel to the forehead during the treatment.

If anal fissures are being treated the time spent in the bath can be up to 30 minutes. For other conditions eight minutes is adequate. At the end of the bath rub the immersed area briefly with a towel that has been wrung out in cold water. If you have prostate problems, hold the damp cold towel between your legs for 10 seconds or so to cool the perineal area between the rectum and the testicles.

In some conditions such as acute cystitis a *neutral sitz bath* is useful. This involves pelvic immersion in water of the same temperature as the body.

Full Baths
These are useful for any of the conditions listed in chapter 9 on aromatic oils, most notably tiredness, anxiety, muscular stiffness, digestive problems, breathing difficulties, skin

problems, menopausal symptoms, headaches, nervous complaints, cellulite and chronic painful conditions such as arthritis and rheumatism. They are contra-indicated only for people whose skin is sensitive or allergic to whatever is being used in the bath.

For more information about therapeutic full baths, see chapter 11.

Jacuzzis and Hot Tubs

If you have access to a hot tub or jacuzzi this can be a help in applying heat to the painful areas of your body, and the underwater jets can apply massage as well, with all the benefits that brings. They are increasingly to be found in health clubs, health centres, in better hotels and in more and more private homes. Many rehabilitation centres and hospitals use whirlpool baths and jacuzzis for treating pain, wounds, skin sores, chronic swellings and specific joint problems such as tennis elbow and arthritic knees. Circulation is also dramatically toned and muscles become more relaxed – and so will you – after a while in these super baths.

After any such hot treatment always apply a short cold treatment (such as a towel wrung out in cold water and briskly rubbed over the skin for 10 seconds or so) to any painful area being treated or to the body as a whole (a short tepid shower would do) to stimulate circulation more. But do not do this if you are aiming only at relaxing. Just dry off, lie down and rest.

Enemas and Colonic Irrigations

These methods, which send water and other fluids to wash out either the lower bowel (enema) or the colon as a whole (colonic irrigation), are extremely useful *when used appropriately.* They should *not* be used as part of your home health-care programme unless recommended by a health-care professional who understands their use and value, because the delicate flora ('friendly bacteria') of the intestinal tract can be severely depleted and damaged if there is unnecessary use of these 'washouts'. There is little danger to health if they are used judiciously, but excessive use of these methods is not a good idea.

When they are used their value is enhanced if the water also contains either herbal products to soothe the mucous membrane of the digestive tract (pure aloe vera juice, for example) or friendly bacteria for re-implantation at the end of the procedure.

Conditions that can be Helped by Water Therapy

This list of conditions is partial – many more can be helped by water therapy. It does not include the use of reflex skin areas as described in chapter 7. When essential oil baths are referred to, the list of oils discussed in chapter 9 should be consulted in order to decide which individual oils or combinations of oils would be best.

Anxiety Neutral bath, stage two of wet-sheet pack, various essential oil baths.
Arthritis Heating compress, fomentations, full sheet pack (all four stages), various essential oil baths, Epsom salts bath, ice pack (if the condition is actively inflamed), alternating sitz baths.
Backache Fomentations, hot sitz bath, heating compress, full sheet pack (all four stages), various essential oil baths, Epsom

salts bath, alternating sitz bath when the back is not in an acute phase.

Bites, stings Ice packs, various essential oil applications/baths.

Bursitis Ice-pack, alternating hot and cold applications, alternating sitz baths.

Breathing problems Various essential oil baths, steam inhalations, heating compress (trunk and chest).

Cellulite Various essential oil baths, local hot and cold applications.

Chest (tight, congested) Heating compress, neutral bath, steam inhalations, alternating sitz baths, Epsom salts bath (if vitality is good), various essential oil baths.

Chest pain (intercostal neuralgia) Fomentations, heating compress, full sheet pack (all stages), neutral bath.

Congestion If chronic use heating compress, fomentations, full sheet pack (all stages), alternating sitz baths. If acute use ice-packs or ice massage, local alternating compresses/applications, full sheet pack (first two stages only).

Constipation Hot sitz bath for atonic constipation, full sheet pack to include stage three for bowel discomfort related to constipation.

Cystitis Neutral sitz bath, various essential oil baths.

Digestive problems Various essential oil baths, full sheet pack (first three stages), heating compress.

Depression Various essential oil baths, full sheet pack (first two stages).

Detoxification Epsom salts bath, full sheet pack (all stages), various essential oil baths, heating compress (on trunk to cover liver area).

Dysmenorrhoea Various essential oil baths, hot sitz bath, fomentations.

Exhaustion (fatigue) Alternating sitz baths, full sheet pack (first stage only for no more than five minutes), various essential oil baths, cold baths as described in chapter 6.

Fever If vitality is good, full sheet pack (first stage only for five minutes or less); to hasten the onset of a fever which is building slowly (if vitality is fair) full sheet pack (all stages); steam inhalations if fever is accompanied by congestion; Epsom salts bath if sweating is needed (five minutes only); heating compress (on trunk) overnight.

Fluid retention Neutral bath (as long an immersion as possible – see chapter 6 on research into this application), full sheet pack (all stages or end after second stage if vitality poor), various essential oil baths (those with diuretic effect – see chapter 9), Epsom salts bath.

Haemorrhoids Alternating sitz baths, ice pack if acute, alternating local applications, hot sitz bath if constipated (use cold application to haemorrhoids after bowels move).

Headache Before it is fully established, mustard foot bath; once established, use various essential oil baths, ice pack, full sheet pack (all stages); if tension headache, neutral bath; if toxic headache, Epsom salts bath.

Heart tonic Neutral bath, full sheet pack (to include stage two), cold bathing according to guidelines given in chapter 6 (if there is a heart condition for which treatment is being given, check with your doctor first).

Inflammation Alternate sitz baths, ice-pack or ice massage, heating compress.

Injuries Heating compress, ice-pack, ice massage, alternating sitz baths, alternating hot and cold applications.

Insomnia Various essential oil baths, full sheet pack (all stages), neutral bath, Epsom salts bath (if vitality is good), heating compress (on abdominal and chest area).

Joint pain/swelling Ice-pack (when acute), heating compress, full sheet pack (all stages, especially if pain is chronic or very acute), various essential oil baths, Epsom salts bath, alternating sitz baths.

Mastitis Heating compress, full sheet pack, hot/cold sitz baths.

Menopausal problems Various essential oil baths, full sheet pack (all stages), neutral bath, cold bathing according to guidelines given in chapter 6.

Muscle aches and spasm Fomentations, full sheet pack (all stages), neutral bath, various essential oil baths, hot sitz bath, ice-pack or ice massage if acute.

Pain Acute or chronic: full sheet pack (all stages), neutral bath, heating compress to local area, Epsom salts bath (if chronic).

Pelvic inflammatory problems Neutral sitz bath if acute, alternating sitz baths if chronic, fomentations, heating compress.

Skin sensitivity and problems Oatmeal bath, fomentations, full sheet pack (first two stages), various essential oil baths, steam treatments (face sauna) for cleansing.

Sinus Steam inhalations, mustard foot bath, hot/cold sitz baths.

Sore throat Heating compress (on throat and trunk simultaneously – two separate compresses at the same time), steam inhalations to decongest, alternating sitz baths.

Sprains Alternating applications, ice massage, ice-pack.

Stress-related tension Various essential oil baths, neutral bath, full sheet pack (all stages or end after stage two).

Toothache Ice pack.

Varicose veins Alternating sitz baths, various essential oil baths for circulation.

Note

- Choose the easiest and most convenient method of application for you.
- Do not use more than one method on any one day.
- To get the best results, some methods (sitz baths, wet sheet packs, compresses, hot/cold local-area bathing) should be repeated every day or two for one to two weeks, especially where the condition is chronic.

13

Exercise – In and Out of Water

There are two key forms of exercise that are important if you are to get the most out of home health and beauty programmes. One involves active movement, using the aerobic principle, and the other involves slow, stretching movements, such as those in yoga and tai chi. One without the other will result in imbalance: to have healthy, 'fit' muscles which are also pliable you need to use both.

Your Aerobic Index

In order to achieve aerobic conditions effectively, and so tone circulation and heart function, you have to exercise neither too strenuously nor too gently. There is a mathematical formula that can tell you how much you need to do to really get the most benefit. Working out your 'aerobic index' is therefore desirable, but it is not essential. If you want to be unstructured in your exercising, without any feeling of having periodically to check your pulse to see whether you are doing 'enough' or 'too much', then forget the formula and just do as much as you want to – it might be all you need. If, however, you want to do what the professionals do, it is certainly the best choice.

The first step is to have a watch with a second hand plus a pencil and paper by your bed to check your resting pulse on waking in the morning. So, before getting up, take your pulse for a full minute and record it. Do the same three mornings running, then add the three numbers together and divide by three to get an average resting pulse rate.

Let's say your resting pulse rate is 70. Add this number to your age. Let's say this is 40.

$$70 + 40 = 110.$$

For reasons which are not important you take that number away from 220.

$$220 - 110 = 110.$$

You are now required to do some serious arithmetic. You need to know what 60% and 80% of the latest figure (110) are.

$$110 \div 10 = 11, \times 6 = 66$$
$$110 \div 10 = 11, \times 8 = 88$$

Now after all this you need to *add back* your morning pulse average.

$$66 + 70 = 136$$
$$88 + 70 = 158$$

These are the magic numbers for aerobics for anyone whose age is 40 and morning resting pulse rate is 70. Remember this is an example only – to find the index you need to apply you must use *your own* resting pulse rate and *your own* age.

When you are exercising you need to check your pulse rate periodically – say every five minutes – to make sure that it stays *above* the lower figure (136 in this example) for 20 minutes not less than three times a week.

It is necessary to keep this going for at least 20 minutes three times a week in order to achieve an aerobic effect which ensures greater fitness and cardiovascular efficiency. And of course you must make sure that your active pulse rate *stays below* 158 (in this same example), so that you avoid any risk to heart function.

When you check your pulse while exercising do so for only 10 seconds and multiply by 6 (to get the rate for a full minute) – if you stop to take your pulse for too long the aerobic effect can be lost.

It isn't surprising that many people can't be bothered to do all this – although once you have done the arithmetic the rest is simple. If you opt simply to get regular exercise without knowing what your pulse is doing, don't feel guilty – we are not all made the same way! But if you *do* choose to follow these guidelines, remember that as you get fitter month by month you need to recheck your morning pulse rate – it might have gone down, meaning that you need to do less to achieve the aerobic effect. And, of course, as you get older the sums need to be done again each year.

What sort of exercise you opt for is up to you. Whether you skip or use a rebounder (mini-trampoline) or dance to jazz music (or ballet) or run or jog or walk or swim or play a competitive sport, it's all the same to your cardiovascular system. Walking is the safest form of exercise, but the most economical in terms of space and time are skipping and rebounding – a couple of minutes of either of these will help to get and keep your muscles toned, although unless you exercise in an aerobic manner, as described above, you will not achieve cardiovascular toning.

Important things to remember about exercise are that:

- the form of exercise should be enjoyable and not a task

- you should be puffing at the end but not exhausted
- to achieve aerobic effects you need to exercise at least three times a week for not less than 20 minutes each time, getting the pulse rate above the magic number without stress while keeping it below the higher number to avoid cardiac strain
- you should *never* hold your breath when exercising – keep your breathing regular, use your diaphragm, and breathe in and out through your mouth if this is more comfortable

Stretching Exercises

Stretching is vital to health. It keeps muscles free, joints mobile, blood and lymph (the body's 'waste disposal' channels) flowing freely, and prevents the likelihood of strains when you are working out more actively. There is an enormous variety of stretching exercises, as anyone who has been to yoga classes will testify.

Try to achieve stretching in all directions without discomfort – forwards, backwards, sideways, twisting, and so on. Your best chance of doing these safely is to go to an exercise class for a while to learn the basics and then apply them at home. Failing this, get a good book on the subject and choose from the selection of exercises described. One example of stretching is given below, from which you can learn the basic rules of *all* safe stretching.

Spinal and Hamstring Stretch

Sit on the floor, on a carpet or your exercise mat, legs straight out in front of you, and bend forwards towards your toes, grasping with your hands the furthest part of your lower legs you can easily reach *without undue strain*. Your head should be hanging as close to your thighs or knees as is comfortably possible. Hold this position for a full minute. While in the position do some slow deep breathing and relax completely. After about six or seven breaths, as you are breathing out stretch a little further down the legs and hold this second position for a further half-minute before slowly sitting up straight.

Next, bend one leg, letting the knee fall to the side, and place the foot against your straight leg near the knee. Bend forwards down the straight leg (when doing stretching exercises always move while you are breathing out) as far as is comfortable and hold the leg with both hands as your head hangs down towards the knee on that side. After a minute of deep breathing, on exhalation, stretch further down the leg and hold for another half-minute. Slowly sit up and change legs so that the one that was bent is now straight and vice versa. Repeat the stretch as described above.

On sitting up again, repeat the stretch with both legs straight, and see how much further you can now go.

Forget the dictum 'no pain, no gain' – there should be no pain on doing stretching exercises. Rather, it should be a pleasant and relaxing experience.

Ten minutes each day devoted to stretching pays dividends, especially if you vary the stretches to cover all possible directions. What's best is to choose half a dozen regular stretches, of which the one above is a useful starter. Enjoy the process – it should not be a burden to you.

Water Exercises

You can do more things in water than out of it, especially if your joints are stiff and achy, because water supports the body more than air does. Obviously a pool is going to provide greater scope than a bath, but there is still much to achieve in a confined space. Any exercise (in or out of water) should be painless and should be performed slowly and deliberately. If you are standing in the bath or shower have a slip mat in place. Have the water you are in warm and the room draught free.

Basic Exercises for the Bath

These exercises are for stiff or painful joints and muscles.

Whatever part is stiff, restricted or uncomfortable should be allowed a few minutes of gentle soaking. Ideally the bath should have some Epsom salts and/or sea salt in it. Gently move the part (knee, ankle, elbow, neck, or even back) in various directions, carefully paying attention to the direction(s) of maximum 'bind' or restriction and the direction(s) of maximum ease. Then try one of the following three exercises. If the first or the second is successful, you can repeat it the next time you bathe. If it isn't, you can use the other exercise next time, or try the third exercise.

Exercise 1

This is most suitable for stiff and restricted parts that are not particularly painful.

Take the joint towards the most restricted position but not to the point of pain. Stay in this position for about 15 seconds and then see whether you can *without force or pain* go a little further towards the restricted direction. If you are successful, repeat until no further gain is possible.

Exercise 2

This is most suitable for areas that are restricted and painful on movement or just painful.

Take the joint towards the direction of maximum ease – where it feels to be most 'free' and unrestricted (take a minute or two to find this position). Hold this for a full minute and then gently see whether you can take it more easily in the previously restricted or painful direction.

Exercise 3

Slowly and deliberately move the joint as far as possible, while it is underwater, in all the directions that are not restricted or painful. Keep moving and repeat the directions that are 'easy', avoiding all painful movements. Do this for two or three minutes before resting. See how the area feels the next day. If it is easier, use this method again.

Aquarobics

To achieve useful levels of toning exercise in water you need access to a swimming pool or the sea. As with all aerobic exercise, always stretch beforehand to 'warm up' the muscles in preparation for what is to come and to avoid injury. Get a book on warm up exercises and do what is appropriate for your needs.

To achieve real toning benefit from water exercise join a class – there is no substitute for an expert leading you. If you want to go it alone in a pool then settle for swimming, or get hold of one of the many books now available on pool exercises. If swimming is what you choose, start with a few lengths or breadths of the pool and gradually train yourself to do as many as you can, using the pulse test to make sure that you are not overdoing it and that you are doing enough to make a difference to your fitness level.

Swimming and Your Neck

Whether you are doing crawl or breast stroke, swimming places a lot of stress on your neck unless your face is in the water. So, whatever it looks like, you might want to avoid this strain by getting yourself swimming goggles or a water-tight face-mask and a snorkel, and swim face down in the water, breathing through the snorkel, and every now and then raising your eyes just enough to see where you are going.

Caution

Stop whatever exercise you are doing if you

- feel tightness or pain in your chest
- become severely breathless
- become lightheaded or dizzy or feel nausea
- feel exhausted
- lose muscle control

Stop and rest, and if the symptom persists call a doctor.

14

Sea and Sun for Health

Sea Water Treatment

Treatment involving sea water or the sea is known as thalassotherapy, which comes from the Greek word *thalassa* meaning 'the sea'. The word was coined in 1867 in France to describe the many therapeutic uses of sea water, sea (beach) sand, sea weed, sea mud, and other substances derived from the sea.

Thalassotherapy includes using sea water for bathing, exercising and even drinking. Unpolluted sea water has unique anti-bacterial effects due to the minute plant-life (plankton) which keeps the sea pure. Pollution can, however, overwhelm this cleansing process and modern thalasso-therapy centres require strict testing for contamination. Sea water can be used internally and externally in all the ways in which water therapy is used, as a means of treating a wide range of ailments or just for keeping fit. The salt content in oceans, which is thought to account for many of the benefits of thalassotherapy, is around 35 grams per litre, rising to 42 grams per litre in the Red Sea and higher still in the Dead Sea.

Sea mud, which contains algae and seaweeds, is used in some thalassotherapy centres to treat skin and rheumatic conditions by being applied to the relevant areas. Similarly, dry or wet beach sand, which contains sea residues, can be used for application of heat, by covering painful joints in hot sand for example.

A variation of thalassotherapy is 'climatotherapy', which involves use of the unique qualities of the air and climate, for example on the north-west coasts of Denmark and Germany. Aerosols are sometimes made of sea water for inhalation to help breathing problems. Similarly, the prevailing sea breezes, which carry sea spray and a high level of health-promoting negative ionisation particles, are used for inhalation.

Modern sea-water treatment centres are custom built with complex pools of varying depth for different uses, various temperatures of water, horizontal and vertical showers, exercise pools, 'walking' pools, special foot and arm bathing areas, and 'mud bath' rooms, rest and drying rooms. Most follow strict hygiene standards, especially in Germany and France, with the water usually being drawn from a safe distance out and at a depth guaranteeing purity. The salt content and radioactivity is monitored and a safe bacterial count maintained. In addition, a variety of tests and precautions are followed, for example in deciding how many patients can attend the facility at any one time. The pipes used are ceramic to avoid metallic contamination, and in France no factories are allowed within 10 kilometres of thalassotherapy centres.

Conditions that Thalassotherapy can Treat

Skin, circulatory, rheumatic and breathing conditions and fluid retention are the most common problems treated at thalassotherapy facilities. Most treatments involve heat from water, mud or sand, or alternating hot and cold applications of these, which are helpful in treating various forms of arthritis. Joint stiffness and injury are improved as the treatment promotes circulatory changes leading to muscle relaxation. Further improvement is gained from specific thalassotherapy exercise programmes.

The content of the water and mud is varied to suit the needs of different skin conditions, for example by the addition of fresh or dried algae and seaweeds.

Treatment at a Thalassotherapy Centre

Depending upon the sophistication of the facility there might be complex treatment areas, or the whole activity might be confined to a simple bathroom. In some facilities 'walking pools' are designed so that the patient can walk into progressively deeper levels of water, always with railings for support, walking, sitting or standing for a prescribed length of time. Exercises might also be prescribed and performed in the pools. Or baths may be given in heated sea water, with exercises being performed either individually or in classes which are supervised.

Following such immersion the patient might receive a 'Scottish' douche, which consists of a high-pressure spray or jet of cold or hot, or alternating, sea water applied for a short time to specific areas to achieve circulatory or reflex effects. After this, treatment in a specialised solarium involves combining exposure to sun (ultra violet) light, infra red (heat) rays, and possibly sea spray or vaporised sea water. Various mud or sand applications might be used on the joints.

In some centres small amounts of sea water, containing various trace elements such as sulfate, magnesium, iodine and other salts, may be prescribed for drinking. For example, water's potassium content might be used to help fluid retention problems, or the fluoride content might be used to help calcium metabolism if this is unbalanced. The water is given diluted, in its natural state, or with a juice for palatability. Amounts are small, one or two tablespoonsful at most to start with, half an hour before a meal, building gradually until four tablespoons are taken three times daily.

Caution

Almost all thalassotherapy facilities are medically run and a full medical history would allow the accurate prescription of methods. *Consumption of sea water as described above, without stringent hygienic precautions, could be dangerous*.

Probably the only absolute contra-indication against the use of the general thalassotherapy methods applies to pregnant women or those who are very frail, who might find the treatment too exhausting.

Where to Find a Thalassotherapy Centre

Tourist Information Boards of European countries such as France (especially the Brittany region), Belgium, Italy, Russia/Ukraine (the Black Sea), Germany and Denmark should be able to provide lists of their major thalassotherapy centres. There are no thalassotherapy centres in the UK, although some spas use sea salt in some treatments.

Sunlight for Health

Heliotherapy is controlled sunbathing – the use of sunlight as a means of treatment or prevention of disease. Historically there are records as far back as the fourth century BC in which sunlight was used to treat disease – healing of skin ulcers, for example – and in Roman times a solarium was a part of every middle-class villa.

In the early twentieth century Swiss doctors developed 'sun cures' for the treatment of external (skin) tuberculosis and forms of tuberculosis that affected bones and the digestive tract, as well as for the treatment of slow-healing wounds. Heliotherapy was also used to enhance the general health of people with pulmonary TB, as well as for prevention – to help children with a family predisposition to tuberculosis, for example. The use of heliotherapy in sanatoria spread worldwide, usually in mountainous, unpolluted regions, until the discovery of drug treatment for tuberculosis. It was the introduction of streptomycin and other drugs in the 1940s and 1950s which led to a decline in the use of heliotherapy for treating TB, although it had never been seen as the total answer to that disease, rather as a valuable accessory to a more general treatment.

A recent dramatic resurgence of drug-resistant strains of the organism that causes TB has occurred throughout the world, creating a serious health menace especially amongst drug addicts and the homeless, where a combination of poor hygiene and malnutrition are likely to be part of the cause. This appearance of drug-resistant forms of the so-called 'white plague' has led to a revival of heliotherapy in those sanatoria that are still functioning.

How Heliotherapy is Applied

In all cases a slow introduction to the sun's rays is important. Where heliotherapy is used as part of a seaside or spa treatment it would typically involve the person being allowed five minutes exposure on the first day, increasing by five to ten minutes daily until between 30 and 60 minutes of sunbathing was achieved daily. In many instances this is accompanied by warm, vaporised sea water being sprayed over the patient at regular intervals.

Where heliotherapy is applied in a sanatorium in the mountains the method differs. At first the patient, wearing swimming clothes and protective glasses and a hat, lies in the shade for short periods each day, for several days. After this, gradual exposure to direct sunlight begins, in such a way as to avoid any reddening of the skin.

A standard Swiss approach was developed at the turn of the century by Dr Rollier, the main pioneer of heliotherapy, and involves five minutes of exposure of the feet only to sunlight on the first sunbathing day. The following day the feet are exposed for 10 minutes and the lower legs for five minutes. The next day the feet receive 15 minutes, the lower legs 10 minutes and the upper legs five minutes. Progressively, over a period of a week, the whole front of the body is exposed in this way, although the face and head are never exposed to direct sunlight. By the time that the feet are receiving 35 minutes of sunlight and the upper trunk 15 minutes, exposure of the back also begins for five minutes. Progressive increases in exposure continue, always avoiding any burning (redness), until three to four hours of winter sun exposure is received daily (between 10 a.m. and 3 p.m.), with two to three hours allowed in the summer (between 7 a.m. and 11 a.m.).

Where local body areas are being treated, say an ulcerative wound or recent operation scar, it is often useful to expose only that part of the body, again by slowly increased amounts of time.

If there are signs of headache, restlessness, fatigue, insomnia or a rise in temperature or pulse rate, then the amount of treatment is undesirable and a change should be made to reduce exposure.

A feeling of increased well-being, improved appetite and enhanced skin tone in patients treated in this way is usually accompanied by improved blood status, showing that the improvement is not just cosmetic. A common report is that pain diminishes, sometimes to a remarkable degree. Wounds heal and coughs may reduce or disappear. Usually improvements are slow and steady as the treatment progresses.

Artificial sunlight, using sophisticated lamps, has increasingly taken the place of real sunlight, largely for economic reasons. This trend has drawbacks as no lamp fully matches true sunlight in providing the full spectrum of rays, nor does the use of lamps allow for the additional benefits of exposure to unpolluted mountain or sea air during the sunbathing.

The length of a stay at a sanatorium providing heliotherapy treatment is, however, uneconomic, since up to eight months is commonly required before patients can be discharged.

Contra-Indications and Concerns

Anyone with kidney disease, ulcerative enteritis, cardiac conditions, skin cancers or lupus erythematosus should avoid heliotherapy.

Modern concerns over increased radiation hazards due to damage to the ozone layer makes care in the use of heliotherapy even more important. This increased danger should not be seen as a complete barrier to heliotherapy where a need exists, but should reinforce the need for gradual acclimatisation as demanded by Dr Rollier's protocol. Careful monitoring of skin changes and avoidance of exposure of the eyes are also essential.

Sun-lamps

Home or health club use of ultra-violet tanning devices is probably unwise because of the risk of skin cancer which excessive exposure to such rays can produce. Being exposed to air and indirect sunlight for a part of each day, rather than actual sun-bathing, is probably the wisest course of action.

Where to Find a Heliotherapy Centre
Because of the ideal climatic and geographical conditions, sanatoria offering heliotherapy are found mainly in the Alpine and other mountainous regions of Switzerland, Austria and Germany.

15

Hydrotherapy at a Spa or Clinic

Home use of water therapy is valuable and safe, but it is not quite the same as the water treatment you would receive in a health spa, where it would probably be combined with other appropriate treatments including osteopathy, physiotherapy, massage, aromatherapy, reflexology and also relaxation and exercise classes and a dietary programme specifically designed for you. Spas usually have custom-built water-treatment facilities ranging from underwater massage to many different forms of contrast and heat baths. In spas around the world, but particularly in Germany, Switzerland, France and Austria, the range and combinations of treatments are simply mind-boggling. So what happens when you go to them?

Health Hydros and Spas

Most people go to spas to relax, lose weight or recharge – they seldom go with specific health complaints, although if there are any they will be taken into account when the treatment programme is being planned. There will be an initial interview or consultation, usually with a medically qualified person, during which the reasons you give for wanting to have a stay at such a place, how long a stay you plan, your medical history and an evaluation of your present level of well-being (including blood pressure and heart function) will be collated so that a programme can be devised to meet your individual needs.

Clearly if you are only going to be there for a few days the programme will be of a general nature – say a light diet plus daily treatments of massage, relaxation and breathing instruction, hydrotherapy (and in some spas osteopathy and/or acupuncture, if this is appropriate), as well as exercise classes. If a longer stay is possible – say a week or more – then the programme can be more precisely targeted at meeting your needs and might involve specific treatments such as dietary or fasting regimes plus an appropriate combination of treatments as above.

The atmosphere at spas is relaxed, with most people spending the days lounging around in dressing-gowns between their appointed treatments or classes and the all-important mealtimes (however light these may be). There are usually additional sporting or recreational activities, which are optional, ranging from art or cooking or flower arranging classes to guided or individual country walks, swimming, yoga, tai chi or badminton. Most people leave spas feeling renewed – and this should be your aim in applying similar methods at home.

Hydrotherapy Clinics

In more specialised hydrotherapy clinics, mainly in Germany, the methods are even more focused and precise, since most people attending them have real and sometimes serious health problems. After several hundred years of experimentation and development the equipment used in modern hydrotherapy units is now highly technical, often computer controlled for accuracy of temperature and method of application. Applications range from specific body parts being exposed to different temperature water at the same time, with rapid contrasts being introduced at precise time intervals, to high-pressure jets being played on particular reflex regions.

Hyperthermia and Serious Illnesses

In recent years the use of hyperthermia, or artificial fever therapy, has evolved – literally extreme heating of the body for particular purposes such as cancer treatment and treatment of infections, including serious ones such as AIDS.

Viruses and bacteria are heat sensitive, some more so than others, and so are cancer cells. For this reason a number of different hydrotherapy methods of heating the body are used to encourage deactivation or death of viruses, bacteria and cancer cells.

In some clinic settings, most notably in Germany, up to eight hours of immersion in hot water (with frequent cool drinks and cool compresses on the head and neck) are used in treating cancer. This is, however, extremely exhausting for the patient, and should not be tried at home.

At Bastyr College, one of America's leading centres for the teaching of hydrotherapy, AIDS patients were recently prescribed a series of 12 hyperthermia baths at 102°F for 40 minutes, twice weekly, in concentrated batches for three weeks at a time, over the course of a year. The HIV virus is known to be heat sensitive – a number of studies have shown that when the core body temperature is raised, by being in water at a temperature of 42°C for 30 minutes or more, there is a 40 per cent deactivation of HIV. The way in which this and other viruses are deactivated by heat, and the best ways of achieving this, continues to attract medical interest and there is little doubt that the method will continue to be refined for treating some forms of infection as well as for treating cancer.

On no account should you attempt hyperthermic treatment on yourself or a member of your family.

Notes
For more information see

Standish, L., 'One year open trial of naturopathic treatment of HIV infection', *Journal of Naturopathic Medicine* 3(1), pp.42–64, 1992.

Martin, L., *et al.,* 'Disinfection and inactivation of human T-lymphotrophic virus-III lymphadenopathy-associated virus', *Journal of Infectious Disease* 152(2), pp.300–403, 1985.

Weatherburn, H., 'Hyperthermia and AIDS treatment', *British Journal of Radiology* 61, pp. 862–3, 1989.

Index